THE ULTIMATE WEIGHT LOSS COMBO: Exploring The Different Strategies For Weight Loss

Addie E. Marker

Table of contents

Conclusion

Introduction

In the relentless pursuit of health, wellness, and vitality, few endeavors loom as prominently on the horizon as the quest for weight loss. It's a journey embarked upon by countless individuals across the globe, each with their own unique motivations and aspirations, and all united by the common desire to shed excess pounds and embrace a healthier, more vibrant life. For many, this journey represents more than a mere physical transformation; it's a voyage of self-discovery, empowerment, and renewed vitality.

Welcome to "THE ULTIMATE WEIGHT LOSS COMBO" In these pages, we embark on an enlightening expedition through the multifaceted landscape of weight loss, uncovering the diverse array of strategies, methods, and philosophies that beckon us towards our healthiest selves. This isn't just another book about losing weight; it's an exploration of the myriad pathways one can take on this transformative journey.

The pursuit of a healthier body isn't one-size-fits-all. It's not about adhering to a rigid set of rules or adhering to a single, dogmatic approach. Rather, it's a dynamic and ever-evolving quest, influenced by science, psychology, culture, and individual preferences. It's about recognizing that each of us is a unique blend of genetics, experiences, and aspirations, and that our path to wellness must be equally unique.

Why "THE ULTIMATE WEIGHT LOSS COMBO" Because it's about embracing the power of diversity and choice. This book is your comprehensive guide to exploring and understanding the kaleidoscope of weight loss strategies available to you. From time-tested dietary approaches to cutting-edge fitness trends, from the mind-body connection to medical interventions when necessary, we leave no stone unturned in our pursuit of knowledge and empowerment.

But it's not just about amassing knowledge; it's about applying it in a way that works for you. The journey towards a healthier you isn't meant to be a grueling odyssey of deprivation and sacrifice. It's an opportunity for self-empowerment, self-discovery, and self-care. By offering you a multitude of strategies, we enable you to build your own ultimate weight loss combo, a unique blend of methods that align with your goals, lifestyle, and desires.

Throughout this journey, we'll delve into the science of weight loss, dispelling myths and misconceptions, while embracing the undeniable truths that underpin success. We'll explore the critical role of nutrition, exercise, and lifestyle choices, guiding you to make informed decisions that lead to lasting change.

But this book is more than just a repository of facts and figures; it's a roadmap to transformation. It's a journey you embark upon with the understanding that change is not only possible but within your grasp. Whether you're just beginning your journey or seeking to break through plateaus, whether you've struggled with your weight for years or are looking to maintain a hard-won victory, this book is your compass, your guide, and your source of inspiration.

You'll find practical tips, meal plans, workout routines, and expert advice to support your efforts. But perhaps most importantly, you'll uncover the mindset and motivation that will sustain you on this transformative path.

"THE ULTIMATE WEIGHT LOSS COMBO" is more than a book; it's an invitation to embark on a personal odyssey that leads not only to a lighter body but to a brighter, more empowered, and more vibrant life. It's a journey that acknowledges the power of choice, celebrates the uniqueness of each individual, and embraces the diversity of strategies available.

So, let's begin. Turn the page, and let's embark together on a voyage of self-discovery, health, and transformation. It's time to explore the different strategies for weight loss and create your own ultimate weight loss combo, a journey that leads to a healthier, happier, and more vibrant you.

Chapter 1: Understanding Weight Loss

1.1 The Science of Weight Gain and Loss

Weight, an enigma that our bodies grapple with daily, stands at the crossroads of health and wellness. It's a subject that touches the lives of millions, if not billions, of people across the globe. For many, it represents a complex equation with multiple variables, each affecting the overall outcome. In this chapter, we embark on a comprehensive exploration into the science behind weight gain and loss, dissecting the physiological and psychological factors that underpin this universal concern.

The Basics of Energy Balance

At the heart of every weight-related journey lies a fundamental concept: energy balance. It's the principle of calories in versus calories out, a basic equation that dictates whether we gain, lose, or maintain weight. When we consume more calories than our bodies expend, we enter a state of surplus, leading to weight gain. Conversely, when we burn more calories than we ingest, we create a deficit, which triggers weight loss.

Understanding this energy balance is the cornerstone of effective weight management. It's akin to maintaining a financial budget; if you consistently spend more than you earn, you accumulate debt, and if you spend less than you earn, you save. In the context of weight, excess calories become stored as fat, primarily in adipose tissue, serving as an energy reserve for times of scarcity, a survival mechanism deeply ingrained in our biology.

Metabolism, the intricate series of biochemical processes within our bodies, acts as the engine governing this balance. Each individual possesses a unique metabolism, influenced by factors such as genetics, age, gender, and muscle mass. Metabolism determines how efficiently we burn calories and, in part, why some individuals seem to effortlessly maintain their weight while others struggle.

Physical activity, another critical component, significantly impacts the calorie expenditure side of the equation. Regular exercise not only burns calories but also boosts metabolic rate, promoting overall health. Factors like genetics and hormones, however, can influence our appetite and how our bodies store calories. For example, insulin plays a dual role, regulating blood sugar levels but also promoting fat storage. Leptin and ghrelin are hormones that affect hunger and satiety. These hormonal influences can complicate the simplicity of energy balance, making weight management a multifaceted challenge.

The Mechanics of Weight Gain

Weight gain occurs when the body stores excess calories as fat. This process, while seemingly straightforward, is influenced by a myriad of factors, both genetic and environmental. Genetics can determine where your body prefers to store fat and how efficiently it does so. Some individuals may have a genetic predisposition to accumulate excess calories as fat in specific areas, such as the abdomen or thighs. Others may possess a genetic resistance to weight gain.

Hormones, the body's chemical messengers, also play a pivotal role in the regulation of weight. Insulin, for example, not only controls blood sugar levels but also encourages fat storage. Leptin, produced by fat cells, signals to the brain when we've had enough to eat, promoting satiety. Ghrelin, on the other hand, stimulates hunger. Hormonal imbalances can disrupt the delicate equilibrium of energy balance, making it challenging to control weight.

Weight Loss as a Scientific Process

The process of weight loss, contrary to popular belief, is grounded in science rather than magic or mystery. It revolves around the concept of creating an energy deficit, wherein you expend more calories than you consume. This deficit prompts your body to tap into its fat reserves for energy, leading to weight loss.

Despite the alluring promise of spot reduction—losing fat from specific areas through targeted exercises—your body adheres to a more holistic approach. When you create a calorie deficit, your body draws from its fat stores as a whole, reducing fat from various areas gradually. While you can tone and strengthen specific muscle groups, you cannot selectively eliminate fat from a single location.

Beyond the scale, it's essential to consider body composition, which refers to the ratio of fat to lean muscle mass in your body. Successful weight loss isn't just about shedding pounds; it's about reducing body fat percentage and preserving lean muscle. This distinction is crucial for long-term health and sustainability, as it ensures that the weight you lose primarily comprises fat rather than muscle.

Beyond the Scale: Non-Scale Victories

As you embark on your weight loss journey, it's vital to remember that success extends beyond the numbers displayed on the scale. Non-scale victories are equally valuable measures of progress. These victories include improved energy levels, enhanced mood, better sleep quality, and increased fitness and strength. Focusing on these achievements reinforces the positive impact of your efforts on your overall well-being.

Furthermore, it's crucial to differentiate between healthy and unhealthy weight loss. Rapid and extreme weight loss methods may yield quick results but can have adverse effects on your health and metabolism in the long run. Sustainable weight loss emphasizes gradual, healthy changes that you can maintain over time. This approach not only promotes better physical health but also supports mental and emotional well-being.

Setting realistic expectations is paramount to a successful weight loss journey. Rapid transformations are the exception rather than the rule, and the path to sustainable change is often characterized by gradual, steady progress. Embracing this journey as an opportunity for self-improvement, self-discovery, and self-care is key. It's not just about reaching a destination; it's about creating lasting, positive change in your life.

In this exploration of "The Science of Weight Gain and Loss," we've ventured deep into the intricate mechanisms governing our bodies' relationship with weight. Armed with this knowledge, you're not only equipped to make informed decisions but also empowered to set realistic goals and embark on a path that leads to a healthier, happier, and more vibrant version of yourself. The journey of understanding the science of weight is the first step toward mastering it, and the road ahead is filled with promise, potential, and the transformation you seek.

1.2 Different Types of Weight Loss

Weight loss methods vary widely, catering to the diverse needs, preferences, and circumstances of individuals seeking to shed excess pounds. In this extensive discussion, we'll explore a comprehensive range of weight loss approaches, from dietary strategies to exercise regimens, lifestyle modifications, and more.

1. Dietary Approaches

- Calorie Restriction: This classic method involves reducing daily caloric intake to create a calorie deficit, the core principle of weight loss.

- Low-Carb Diets: Including the ketogenic and Atkins diets, these plans restrict carbohydrate consumption while promoting fats and proteins as primary energy sources.

- Low-Fat Diets: These diets prioritize reduced dietary fat intake, emphasizing carbohydrates and lean proteins.

- Plant-Based and Vegetarian Diets: Focusing on whole, plant-based foods while minimizing or eliminating animal products.

- Intermittent Fasting: Involving cycles of fasting and eating during specific time windows or days, helping control calorie intake.

- Mediterranean Diet: Emphasizing heart-healthy fats, whole grains, lean proteins, and an abundance of fruits and vegetables.

2. Exercise and Physical Activity

- Cardiovascular Exercise: Activities like running, swimming, cycling, and aerobics elevate heart rate and calorie expenditure, promoting weight loss.

- Strength Training: Building muscle mass through weightlifting, bodyweight exercises, and resistance training boosts metabolism and fat loss.

- Yoga and Mindful Movement: These practices improve balance, flexibility, and mental well-being, complementing weight loss efforts.

- High-Intensity Interval Training (HIIT): Involving short bursts of intense exercise followed by brief rest periods, a time-efficient method for calorie burning.

- Dance and Fun Workouts: Engaging in enjoyable activities like dancing, Zumba, or group fitness classes makes exercise more enjoyable.

- Outdoor Activities: Incorporating outdoor adventures and sports offers exercise combined with enjoyment of nature.

3. Lifestyle Modifications

- Sleep and Weight Loss: The impact of quality sleep on appetite regulation, hormones, and overall weight management.

- Stress Management: Techniques for reducing stress, which can lead to emotional eating and hinder weight loss efforts.

- Mindful Eating and Portion Control: Cultivating awareness of eating habits and controlling portion sizes to prevent overconsumption.

- Habits and Behavioral Changes: Identifying and modifying habits that influence eating and physical activity choices.

- Support Systems and Accountability: The importance of social support, accountability partners, and community for successful weight loss maintenance.

4. Medical and Surgical Approaches

- Bariatric Surgery Options: Surgical interventions like gastric bypass and sleeve gastrectomy for individuals with severe obesity.

- Prescription Medications: Medications prescribed by healthcare professionals to aid in weight loss by suppressing appetite or reducing fat absorption.

- Liposuction and Cosmetic Procedures: Surgical and non-surgical methods for fat reduction and body contouring.

5. Mind-Body Connection

- Mindful Eating and Intuitive Eating: Practices that promote mindful, intuitive approaches to eating, fostering a healthy relationship with food.

- Emotional Eating and Coping Strategies: Recognizing emotional triggers for overeating and developing healthy coping mechanisms.

- Visualization and Affirmations: Techniques for creating positive mental associations with weight loss goals.

- Meditation and Stress Reduction: Mindfulness and relaxation practices to reduce stress-related weight gain.

6. Combining Strategies for Success

- Creating a Personalized Weight Loss Plan: Tailoring strategies to individual preferences, goals, and needs for a more effective approach.

- Tracking Progress and Adjusting Strategies: Monitoring weight loss milestones and adapting approaches as needed for continued success.

- Breaking Through Plateaus: Strategies to overcome weight loss plateaus and maintain progress.

- Setting Realistic Goals: The importance of setting achievable and sustainable weight loss goals for long-term success.

7. Maintaining Weight Loss

- Transitioning to Maintenance Mode: Shifting from active weight loss to weight maintenance, emphasizing long-term health.

- Long-Term Healthy Habits: Strategies for sustaining a healthy lifestyle beyond initial weight loss, promoting overall well-being.

- Preventing Weight Regain: Tips to avoid regaining lost weight and maintaining progress achieved.

8. Celebrating Your Success

- Recognizing Milestones: Celebrating achievements, no matter how small, along the weight loss journey to stay motivated.

- Staying Motivated and Inspired: Finding ongoing inspiration and motivation for maintaining a healthier lifestyle.

- Inspiring Others: Encouraging and supporting others on their weight loss journeys by sharing experiences and knowledge.

By exploring these diverse weight loss methods, individuals can identify the approach that best aligns with their goals and preferences, fostering a sustainable and transformative journey toward a healthier life.

1.3 The Role of Genetics

Weight management, a journey undertaken by millions worldwide, is a complex interplay of various factors. While diet and exercise play pivotal roles in determining our weight, genetics, an inherent aspect of our biology, also exerts a profound influence. The debate on whether genetics predetermine our weight or merely influence it continues to captivate researchers and individuals striving for healthier lives. In this extensive exploration, we delve into the intricate relationship between genetics and weight loss.

Genetics: The Blueprint of Life

Genetics, the study of heredity and the variation of inherited traits, encompasses the genes and DNA sequences passed down from one generation to the next. These genetic instructions shape our physical attributes, susceptibility to diseases, and, to a certain extent, our predisposition to gain or lose weight.

The Genetic Basis of Weight

Genes related to weight regulation can be broadly categorized into two groups: those that influence appetite and metabolism and those that determine body fat distribution.

Appetite and Metabolism Genes: Several genes are associated with appetite control and metabolism regulation. For example, the FTO gene has gained considerable attention in obesity research. Variations in the FTO gene are linked to increased food intake and a higher risk of obesity. Additionally, genes like MC4R (melanocortin-4 receptor) play a role in appetite regulation. Variants in these genes can lead to heightened hunger and cravings, making it more challenging to maintain a calorie deficit for weight loss.

Body Fat Distribution Genes: Genetics also influence where your body tends to store fat. Some individuals may have a genetic predisposition to store excess fat in the abdominal area, known as central or visceral fat, which is associated with a higher risk of metabolic problems. Others may predominantly store fat in the hips and thighs, referred to as peripheral or subcutaneous fat. While genetics play a role in determining fat distribution, lifestyle factors also contribute significantly.

The Heritability of Weight

The concept of heritability measures the extent to which genetic factors contribute to a specific trait or condition. In the case of body weight, studies estimate that genetic factors may account for approximately 40-70% of the variation in body mass index (BMI) among individuals. This variation indicates that while genetics play a substantial role, environmental and lifestyle factors also significantly impact weight.

Interactions Between Genetics and Environment

It's crucial to recognize that genetics do not operate in isolation; they interact with environmental factors to influence weight. These interactions can be complex and vary from person to person. Environmental factors, such as diet, physical activity, sleep, stress, and socioeconomic status, all contribute to the interplay between genes and weight.

Gene-Environment Interaction in Appetite: An individual with genetic variants associated with heightened appetite may be more susceptible to overeating in an environment rich in calorie-dense, readily available foods. Conversely, in an environment that supports healthy eating habits and portion control, genetic predispositions may have a less pronounced effect.

Gene-Environment Interaction in Physical Activity: Genetics can also influence one's inclination toward physical activity. Some individuals may have a genetic predisposition to enjoy and excel in certain sports or physical activities. Conversely, others may have genetic factors that make them more prone to sedentary behaviors. However, environmental factors, such as access to fitness facilities and opportunities for physical activity, significantly affect how genetics manifest in this regard.

The Impact of Epigenetics

Epigenetics is a fascinating field that explores how environmental factors can modify gene expression without altering the underlying DNA sequence. These modifications, which can be passed down to future generations, have implications for weight management. Epigenetic changes can be influenced by factors such as diet, exercise, and stress. For instance, a study found that maternal nutrition during pregnancy can lead to epigenetic changes that affect a child's propensity for obesity later in life.

Genetics and Weight Loss Response

Individuals often wonder whether their genetic makeup affects their response to weight loss efforts. Research suggests that genetics can indeed influence how individuals respond to different weight loss interventions.

1. Dietary Response: Some studies have indicated that individuals with certain genetic variants may respond differently to specific diets. For example, one's genetic profile may make them more responsive to a low-carbohydrate diet, while others may benefit more from a low-fat or balanced diet. Personalized nutrition based on genetic testing is an emerging area of research and application.

2. Exercise Response: Genetics can also impact how individuals respond to exercise in terms of weight loss and fitness improvements. Some may experience more significant weight loss and muscle gain with specific exercise regimens based on their genetic

predisposition for muscle development and metabolic responses.

3. Appetite Regulation: Genetic factors influencing appetite and satiety can play a role in an individual's ability to adhere to a calorie-restricted diet. Those with genetic variants linked to increased hunger may find it more challenging to maintain a reduced calorie intake.

The Genetic Limitation Myth

It's essential to dispel a common misconception: genetics do not equate to an unchangeable destiny when it comes to weight management. While genetic factors can influence weight, they do not preclude individuals from achieving meaningful weight loss and improved health. The interplay of genetics and lifestyle factors provides numerous opportunities for individuals to make positive changes.

Practical Implications

Understanding the role of genetics in weight loss can inform personalized approaches to achieve and maintain a healthy weight. Here are some practical implications:

1. Tailored Approaches: Recognize that what works for one person may not work as effectively for another due to genetic differences. Tailor your weight loss strategy to your unique genetic predispositions and responses.

2. Lifestyle Modification: Embrace a holistic approach that combines genetics-aware dietary choices, exercise routines, and stress management techniques.

3. Professional Guidance: Consider seeking guidance from healthcare professionals and genetic counselors who can provide insights into your

genetic makeup and its relevance to your weight management journey.

4. Sustainability: Focus on sustainable lifestyle changes rather than quick-fix diets. Sustainable changes can override certain genetic predispositions and promote long-term success.

5. Behavioral Strategies: Incorporate behavioral strategies, such as mindfulness and habit formation, to help counteract genetic factors that may influence appetite and eating behaviors.

Genetics undeniably play a significant role in weight management, influencing factors such as appetite, metabolism, and body fat distribution. However, genetics do not dictate an unalterable path to weight gain or loss.

Chapter 2: Nutrition Strategies

2.1 Calorie Counting and Portion Control

In the quest for weight loss and overall health improvement, understanding the principles of calorie counting and portion control is paramount. These fundamental concepts serve as the cornerstones of many successful weight management strategies. In this comprehensive exploration, we delve into the intricate relationship between calorie counting, portion control, and effective weight loss.

The Calorie Conundrum

Calories, units of energy derived from the food we consume, play a pivotal role in determining our body weight. The basic principle of weight management is to maintain a balance between the number of calories we consume and the number we expend. To lose weight, we need to create a calorie deficit, expending more calories than we ingest. Conversely, to gain weight, we must consume more calories than we burn. Calorie counting is the practice of tracking and quantifying the caloric content of the foods we eat to achieve our desired weight goals.

Calorie Counting: The Science Behind It

1. Understanding Basal Metabolic Rate (BMR): Every individual has a unique BMR, the number of calories the body requires to maintain basic functions while at rest. BMR is influenced by factors such as age, gender, weight, and muscle mass. Calorie counting begins by calculating your BMR, providing a baseline for your daily caloric needs.

2. Determining Total Daily Energy Expenditure (TDEE): To account for physical activity, you must calculate your TDEE, which includes the calories burned through daily activities and exercise. Your daily caloric intake should be adjusted based on your activity level.

3. Setting a Caloric Deficit: Weight loss occurs when you consume fewer calories than your TDEE. A common guideline is to create a calorie deficit of 500 to 1,000 calories per day to lose about 1 to 2 pounds per week, a safe and sustainable rate of weight loss.

The Benefits of Calorie Counting

1. Precision: Calorie counting offers a precise method for tracking and controlling your calorie intake. This precision allows you to fine-tune your weight loss efforts according to your goals.

2. Awareness: Tracking calories raises awareness of your eating habits, helping you identify areas where you may be consuming excess calories. It encourages mindful eating and promotes healthier food choices.

3. Accountability: Calorie counting holds you accountable for your dietary choices. When you track what you eat, you're less likely to underestimate your calorie intake or overlook high-calorie foods.

4. Flexible Choices: Calorie counting doesn't restrict your food choices; it merely guides you in making informed decisions. You can enjoy a variety of foods while still meeting your calorie goals.

Portion Control: Size Matters

Portion control complements calorie counting by managing the quantity of food you consume. It involves moderating portion sizes to align with your calorie goals, ensuring that you eat an appropriate amount of food without overindulging.

The Science Behind Portion Control

1. Perception vs. Reality: The human brain can be easily influenced by external cues, such as plate size and portion size. We often consume what is in front of us, irrespective of our actual hunger levels. Portion control helps bridge the gap between perception and reality.

2. Sensory Satisfaction: Controlling portion sizes can enhance your sensory satisfaction with a meal. Eating slowly and savoring smaller portions can lead to a sense of fullness and satisfaction, even with fewer calories.

3. Digestive Efficiency: Smaller portions are more efficiently digested and absorbed by the body. This can help regulate blood sugar levels and reduce the risk of overeating.

The Benefits of Portion Control

1. Preventing Overeating: Portion control helps prevent the consumption of excess calories, a common contributor to weight gain. By moderating portion sizes, you're less likely to consume more calories than your body needs.

2. Mindful Eating: Practicing portion control encourages mindful eating, which involves paying attention to the sensory experience of eating. This mindfulness can reduce emotional eating and promote healthier relationships with food.

3. Sustainable Habits: Portion control fosters sustainable eating habits that can

be maintained over the long term. It promotes balance and moderation in your diet, which is key to sustained weight management.

4. Calorie Counting and Portion Control: A Synergistic Approach while calorie counting and portion control are valuable tools on their own, their combination offers a powerful approach to weight loss and maintenance. Here's how they work together synergistically:

5. Precision with Portion Control: Calorie counting provides the precision needed to track your daily caloric intake accurately. By knowing how many calories are in each portion of food, you can adjust your portion sizes to meet your calorie goals effectively.

6. Mindful Eating: Portion control encourages mindful eating by helping you become more aware of portion sizes and your body's hunger cues. When

paired with calorie counting, it's easier to make informed choices and resist the temptation to overeat.

7.   Flexibility: Combining calorie counting and portion control allows for greater flexibility in your diet. You can enjoy a wider range of foods while still adhering to your calorie targets.

8. Sustainable Lifestyle: Together, these practices contribute to the development of sustainable lifestyle habits. By mastering portion control and calorie awareness, you're better equipped to maintain a healthy weight in the long term.

Practical Tips for Calorie Counting and Portion Control

1. Use Measuring Tools: Invest in measuring cups, a kitchen scale, and other tools to accurately measure portions.

2. Read Labels: Pay attention to food labels to determine the calorie content and serving size.

3. Keep a Food Journal: Tracking your daily food intake in a journal or mobile app can help you stay accountable.

4. Practice Mindfulness: Eat slowly, savor each bite, and pay attention to hunger and fullness cues.

2.2 Low-Carb, High-Protein Diets

Low-carb, high-protein diets have garnered significant attention in recent years as effective weight loss strategies and means to promote overall health. These dietary approaches center on reducing carbohydrate intake while increasing protein consumption. In this extensive discussion, we delve into the intricacies of low-carb, high-protein diets, examining their principles, potential benefits, considerations, and long-term implications.

The Foundation of Low-Carb, High-Protein Diets

Low-carb, high-protein diets are characterized by a fundamental shift in macronutrient distribution, primarily reducing carbohydrates while increasing protein and, often, dietary fat. The core principles include:

1. Carbohydrate Restriction: These diets emphasize limiting or avoiding high-carb foods such as grains, sugary items, starchy vegetables, and many processed foods. Carbohydrates are replaced with protein and, in some cases, healthy fats.

2. Protein Emphasis: High-quality protein sources, including lean meats,

poultry, fish, eggs, dairy, legumes, and plant-based alternatives, take center stage in these diets. Protein is the primary macronutrient that provides energy and supports muscle growth and maintenance.

3. Reduced Sugar Intake: Sugar intake is significantly curtailed or eliminated to control blood sugar levels and reduce cravings.

4. Increased Healthy Fats: While not all low-carb, high-protein diets prioritize fat intake, some versions allow for moderate to high healthy fat consumption from sources like avocados, nuts, seeds, and olive oil.

The Science Behind Low-Carb, High-Protein Diets

The success of low-carb, high-protein diets is often attributed to several physiological mechanisms:

1. Reduced Insulin Levels: Carbohydrate restriction lowers insulin levels in the body. Insulin, a hormone responsible for storing excess glucose as fat, plays a key role in fat storage. Lower insulin levels are thought to promote fat breakdown and weight loss.

2. Appetite Regulation: High-protein intake has been shown to enhance feelings of fullness and reduce appetite, leading to lower calorie intake.

3. Thermogenesis: Protein has a higher thermogenic effect than carbohydrates or fats, meaning the body expends more energy (calories) to metabolize and digest protein. This can contribute to increased calorie expenditure.

4. Muscle Preservation: Protein is essential for preserving lean muscle mass, which is particularly important

during weight loss to maintain metabolic rate and overall health.

Potential Benefits of Low-Carb, High-Protein Diets

1. Weight Loss: Low-carb, high-protein diets have demonstrated effectiveness in promoting weight loss, often in the short term. The reduction in carbohydrates can lead to decreased water retention and initial weight loss, followed by fat loss as the body adjusts to using stored fat for energy.

2. Improved Blood Sugar Control: Carbohydrate restriction can help stabilize blood sugar levels, making low-carb diets appealing to individuals with type 2 diabetes or those at risk.

3. Enhanced Appetite Control: The satiating nature of protein-rich foods can reduce hunger and cravings, making

it easier to adhere to a calorie-restricted diet.

4. Better Triglyceride Levels: Some studies suggest that low-carb diets can lead to improved triglyceride levels, reducing the risk of heart disease.

5. Positive Impact on HDL Cholesterol: High-protein, low-carb diets may increase high-density lipoprotein (HDL) cholesterol, often referred to as "good" cholesterol.

Considerations and Potential Drawbacks

While low-carb, high-protein diets offer several benefits, they also come with considerations and potential drawbacks:

1. Nutrient Balance: Restricting carbohydrates can sometimes lead to insufficient fiber and essential nutrients. Careful planning is required to ensure

adequate intake of vitamins, minerals, and dietary fiber.

2. Ketosis Risk: Extremely low-carb diets may induce ketosis, a metabolic state where the body burns fat for energy. While some people intentionally aim for ketosis, it's not suitable for everyone and should be approached with caution.

3. Gastrointestinal Issues: High protein intake can lead to digestive discomfort, such as constipation or diarrhea, if not balanced with fiber-rich foods and sufficient fluid intake.

4. Long-Term Sustainability: Low-carb, high-protein diets may be challenging to sustain over the long term due to potential monotony and social limitations.

5. Kidney Function: Individuals with pre-existing kidney conditions should

exercise caution with high-protein diets, as they may place additional strain on the kidneys.

6. Cholesterol Levels: While some people experience improved cholesterol profiles on low-carb diets, others may see unfavorable changes, such as increased LDL cholesterol. Individual responses can vary.

Balancing Low-Carb, High-Protein Diets for Success

To optimize the benefits of low-carb, high-protein diets while mitigating potential drawbacks, consider the following guidelines:

1. Choose Quality Protein: Opt for lean sources of protein such as poultry, fish, legumes, and plant-based alternatives.

2. Incorporate Non-Starchy Vegetables: Include a variety of non-starchy

vegetables to provide essential nutrients and fiber while keeping carb intake in check.

3. Monitor Portion Sizes: Pay attention to portion control to avoid excessive calorie intake.

4. Stay Hydrated: Adequate fluid intake is crucial to prevent dehydration, especially when reducing carbohydrate intake.

5. Include Healthy Fats: Incorporate sources of healthy fats like avocados, nuts, seeds, and olive oil for balanced nutrition.

6. Consult a Professional: Before embarking on a low-carb, high-protein diet, consult with a healthcare professional or registered dietitian to ensure it aligns with your health goals and individual needs.

Low-carb, high-protein diets offer a structured approach to weight loss and improved metabolic health. When implemented with care, these diets can lead to positive outcomes, including weight loss, better blood sugar control, and enhanced appetite regulation. However, they may not be suitable for everyone, and individual responses vary. It's essential to approach any dietary change with mindfulness, emphasizing nutrient balance, sustainability, and overall health as primary goals. Consulting a healthcare professional or dietitian can provide personalized guidance for success on a low-carb, high-protein diet.

2.3 Plant-Based and Vegetarian Diets

Plant-based and vegetarian diets have gained immense popularity in recent years, not only for their ethical and environmental considerations but also for their potential benefits in promoting weight loss and overall health. These diets emphasize whole, plant-derived foods while excluding or minimizing animal products. In this comprehensive discussion, we explore the principles, potential advantages, considerations, and strategies for successful weight loss with plant-based and vegetarian diets.

The Essence of Plant-Based and Vegetarian Diets

Plant-based and vegetarian diets are distinguished by their emphasis on plant-derived foods, including fruits, vegetables, legumes, whole grains, nuts, and seeds. The extent of animal product exclusion varies:

1. Plant-Based Diet: Primarily consists of plant foods and may occasionally include small amounts of animal products. Some plant-based diets exclude all animal products, while others permit occasional consumption of dairy, eggs, or fish.

2. Vegetarian Diet: Excludes all meat, poultry, and seafood but may include dairy and eggs. There are different types of vegetarian diets, such as lacto-vegetarian (includes dairy) and ovo-vegetarian (includes eggs).

The Science Behind Plant-Based and Vegetarian Diets

Numerous studies have explored the potential health benefits of plant-based and vegetarian diets, particularly in the context of weight management. Here are some key scientific principles:

1. Lower Calorie Density: Plant-based foods, such as fruits, vegetables, and legumes, are generally lower in calorie density compared to animal products and processed foods. This can promote weight loss by allowing individuals to consume larger portions with fewer calories.

2. High Fiber Content: Plant-based diets are rich in dietary fiber, which contributes to feelings of fullness and satiety. Fiber also slows down digestion, stabilizing blood sugar levels and reducing post-meal cravings.

3. Reduced Saturated Fat: Plant-based diets typically contain lower levels of saturated fat found in animal products, which can contribute to weight loss and improved heart health.

4. Nutrient Density: Plant-based diets offer a wide array of essential nutrients, vitamins, minerals, and antioxidants,

promoting overall health and vitality during weight loss.

Advantages of Plant-Based and Vegetarian Diets for Weight Loss

1. Weight Loss: Numerous studies suggest that plant-based and vegetarian diets can be effective for weight loss. Reduced calorie intake, improved satiety, and a focus on whole, unprocessed foods contribute to these outcomes.

2. Heart Health: These diets are associated with lower levels of cholesterol and blood pressure, reducing the risk of heart disease, a common concern for those seeking weight loss.

3. Improved Metabolic Health: Plant-based diets may enhance insulin sensitivity and reduce the risk of type 2 diabetes.

4. Digestive Health: High fiber intake supports healthy digestion and can alleviate issues such as constipation.

5. Long-Term Sustainability: Many individuals find plant-based and vegetarian diets to be sustainable and enjoyable, increasing the likelihood of long-term adherence.

Considerations and Potential Drawbacks

While plant-based and vegetarian diets offer numerous advantages, they also present considerations and potential challenges:

1. Nutrient Balance: Proper planning is essential to ensure adequate intake of nutrients such as protein, vitamin B12, iron, zinc, and omega-3 fatty acids, which can be limited in plant-based diets.

2. Variety: Ensuring dietary variety is crucial to prevent monotony and to obtain a wide spectrum of nutrients.

3. Social and Cultural Factors: Social situations and cultural practices can sometimes pose challenges for individuals adhering to plant-based or vegetarian diets.

4. Nutritional Education: Those new to plant-based or vegetarian eating may benefit from nutritional guidance to meet their dietary needs.

5. Potential for Processed Foods: While plant-based diets emphasize whole foods, it's possible to rely on highly processed, plant-based alternatives that may not support weight loss goals.

Strategies for Successful Weight Loss with Plant-Based and Vegetarian Diets

1. Balanced Meals: Focus on balanced meals that incorporate a variety of plant-based foods, including vegetables, fruits, whole grains, legumes, nuts, and seeds.

2. Protein Sources: Include plant-based protein sources such as tofu, tempeh, seitan, legumes, and quinoa in your diet to meet protein needs.

3. Nutrient Monitoring: Pay attention to nutrient intake, particularly vitamin B12, iron, calcium, and omega-3 fatty acids. Consider supplementation or fortified foods as needed.

4. Portion Control: Be mindful of portion sizes, even with plant-based foods. Overeating can hinder weight loss progress.

5. Limit Processed Foods: Minimize the consumption of highly processed

plant-based foods, which may be calorie-dense and less filling.

6. Hydration: Stay adequately hydrated with water and herbal teas to support digestion and reduce the risk of mistaking thirst for hunger.

7. Consultation: Consider consulting a registered dietitian or nutritionist for personalized guidance and meal planning.

Plant-based and vegetarian diets offer a holistic approach to weight loss, promoting overall health, and supporting sustainable dietary choices. Their emphasis on whole, plant-derived foods aligns with principles that have been linked to weight loss success, including lower calorie density, high fiber content, reduced saturated fat intake, and nutrient density. However, it's essential to approach these diets with careful planning and nutritional awareness to ensure nutrient balance. With proper consideration and education, plant-based and vegetarian diets can be effective and enjoyable pathways to achieving weight loss and long-term well-being.

2.4 Intermittent Fasting

Intermittent fasting (IF) has surged in popularity as a weight loss strategy and lifestyle choice. This dietary approach alternates between periods of fasting and eating, with the primary goal of achieving various health benefits, including weight loss. In this comprehensive discussion, we will delve into the principles, potential advantages, considerations, and strategies for successful weight loss with intermittent fasting.

Understanding Intermittent Fasting

Intermittent fasting is not defined by the types of foods you eat but by when you eat them. It involves cycles of fasting, where you refrain from caloric consumption, followed by eating periods. There are several common methods of intermittent fasting:

1. The 16/8 Method: This method involves fasting for 16 hours and limiting eating to an 8-hour window each day. For instance, you might eat between 12:00 PM and 8:00 PM, fasting from 8:00 PM to 12:00 PM the following day.

2. The 5:2 Method: In this approach, you consume your regular diet five days a week and significantly restrict calorie intake (usually around 500-600 calories) on the other two non-consecutive days.

3. The Eat-Stop-Eat Method: With this method, you fast for a full 24 hours once or twice a week, refraining from any calorie intake during the fasting period.

4. The Alternate-Day Fasting Method: Alternate-day fasting alternates between days of regular eating and days of fasting or consuming very few calories.

5. The Warrior Diet: This method involves eating small amounts of raw fruits and vegetables during the day and having one large meal in the evening, often within a 4-hour eating window.

The Science Behind Intermittent Fasting

Intermittent fasting triggers various physiological changes in the body that can contribute to weight loss and overall health:

1. Caloric Restriction: Intermittent fasting typically leads to a reduced caloric intake over time, creating a calorie deficit necessary for weight loss.

2. Insulin Sensitivity: Fasting periods can improve insulin sensitivity, helping the body use glucose more efficiently and potentially reducing the risk of type 2 diabetes.

3. Fat Utilization: During fasting, the body may shift from primarily using glucose for energy to utilizing stored fat, contributing to fat loss.

4. Autophagy: Intermittent fasting may stimulate autophagy, a cellular process that removes damaged or dysfunctional components, potentially promoting cellular health.

5. Hormonal Changes: Fasting can lead to changes in hormones like growth hormone and norepinephrine, which

can support fat breakdown and metabolism.

Potential Advantages of Intermittent Fasting for Weight Loss

1. Effective Weight Loss: Intermittent fasting has been shown in various studies to be effective for weight loss, often comparable to continuous calorie restriction diets.

2. Simplicity: Intermittent fasting can be straightforward and doesn't require complex meal planning or calorie counting.

3. Flexible and Sustainable: Many people find intermittent fasting to be flexible and sustainable, as it can be adapted to fit individual schedules and preferences.

4. Metabolic Health: Improved insulin sensitivity and other metabolic changes may enhance overall health and reduce the risk of obesity-related diseases.

5. Appetite Control: Some individuals experience reduced appetite during fasting periods, making it easier to maintain a calorie deficit.

Considerations and Potential Drawbacks

1. Hunger and Cravings: Fasting periods can lead to hunger and cravings, which may be challenging for some individuals to manage.

2. Adaptation Period: It may take time for the body to adapt to intermittent fasting, and some people may experience initial discomfort.

3. Nutrient Intake: It's essential to pay attention to nutrient intake during

eating periods to ensure a balanced diet and adequate micronutrient consumption.

4. Individual Variability: Intermittent fasting may not be suitable for everyone, and individual responses can vary widely.

5. Social and Lifestyle Factors: Social events and daily routines can sometimes clash with fasting schedules, requiring adjustment and flexibility.

Strategies for Successful Intermittent Fasting for Weight Loss

1. Choose the Right Method: Select an intermittent fasting method that aligns with your lifestyle, preferences, and daily routine.

2. Stay Hydrated: Drink plenty of water during fasting periods to stay hydrated.

3. Prioritize Nutrient-Dense Foods: Consume nutrient-dense foods, such as fruits, vegetables, lean proteins, and whole grains, during eating windows.

4. Monitor Hunger Signals: Pay attention to your body's hunger signals and adjust your fasting schedule or meal size accordingly.

5. Gradual Adjustment: If new to intermittent fasting, consider gradually increasing fasting durations to allow your body to adapt.

6. Consult a Professional: Consult with a healthcare professional or registered dietitian before starting intermittent fasting, especially if you have underlying health conditions or concerns.

Intermittent fasting is a popular and potentially effective approach to weight loss that emphasizes when you eat rather than what you eat. With its various methods, it offers flexibility and simplicity, making it an attractive choice for many individuals. While intermittent fasting can lead to weight loss and metabolic improvements, it may not suit everyone, and adherence can vary. It's crucial to approach intermittent fasting with awareness, ensuring nutrient balance and personal suitability. Consulting a healthcare professional or dietitian can provide tailored guidance for incorporating intermittent fasting into your weight loss journey and overall health goals.

2.5 Ketogenic Diet

The ketogenic diet, commonly referred to as the keto diet, has gained significant popularity as a weight loss strategy in recent years. It's a low-carbohydrate, high-fat diet designed to shift your body's metabolism into a state called ketosis, where it primarily burns fat for energy instead of carbohydrates. This dietary approach involves specific food choices that are crucial for achieving and maintaining ketosis. In this comprehensive discussion, we'll explore the foods involved in the ketogenic diet for weight loss in detail.

1. Healthy Fats:

Healthy fats form the foundation of the ketogenic diet. These fats provide the majority of your daily calorie intake and are essential for maintaining ketosis.

- Avocados: These green gems are packed with monounsaturated fats, fiber, and various vitamins and minerals.

- Olive Oil: Extra virgin olive oil is a staple source of healthy fats, rich in antioxidants and anti-inflammatory properties.

- Coconut Oil: A unique source of medium-chain triglycerides (MCTs), which can be rapidly converted into ketones, making it a valuable addition to keto recipes.

- Nuts and Seeds: Almonds, walnuts, chia seeds, and flaxseeds are excellent sources of healthy fats, protein, and fiber.

2. High-Quality Proteins:

While protein intake is moderate on the ketogenic diet, it's essential for maintaining muscle mass and overall health.

- Fatty Fish: Salmon, mackerel, and sardines provide both protein and heart-healthy omega-3 fatty acids.

- Poultry: Chicken and turkey are lean protein options suitable for the keto diet.

- Meat: Beef, pork, lamb, and other meats are rich in protein and can be incorporated into a variety of keto recipes.

- Eggs: Eggs are versatile and nutritious, offering an excellent source of protein.

3. Low-Carb Vegetables:

Although vegetables contain carbohydrates, there are several low-carb options that fit well within the ketogenic diet.

- Leafy Greens: Spinach, kale, Swiss chard, and collard greens are low in carbs and high in vitamins and minerals.

- Cruciferous Vegetables: Broccoli, cauliflower, Brussels sprouts, and cabbage are keto-friendly choices packed with fiber and nutrients.

- Zucchini, Asparagus, and Green Beans: These veggies have relatively low carb content compared to starchier options like potatoes and carrots.

4. Dairy Products:

Full-fat dairy products are encouraged on the keto diet due to their fat content and lower carbohydrate levels.

- Butter: Used for cooking and flavoring dishes.

- Cheese: Varieties like cheddar, mozzarella, and cream cheese are keto-friendly.

- Heavy Cream: A rich addition to keto-friendly sauces and coffee.

- Greek Yogurt: Choose full-fat, plain Greek yogurt without added sugars.

5. Keto-Friendly Sweeteners:

If you have a sweet tooth, there are keto-approved sweeteners that can satisfy your cravings without spiking blood sugar levels.

- Stevia: A natural, calorie-free sweetener.

- Erythritol: A sugar alcohol with minimal impact on blood sugar.

- Monk Fruit Sweetener: Derived from monk fruit, it's another low-calorie, natural sweetener option.

6. Berries (in moderation):

Some berries can be incorporated into the keto diet due to their relatively low carbohydrate and high fiber content.

- Strawberries, Blueberries, and Raspberries: Enjoy these in moderation as a sweet treat.

7. Herbs and Spices:

Seasoning your keto meals with herbs and spices is a fantastic way to add flavor without adding carbs.

- Basil, Oregano, Thyme, Turmeric, Cinnamon: These seasonings can enhance the taste of your dishes.

The ketogenic diet for weight loss is based on a significant reduction in carbohydrate intake and an increase in healthy fats and moderate protein. While it can lead to initial weight loss and other potential health benefits, it's important to consider factors like sustainability, potential side effects (e.g., "keto flu"), and individual variability. Consulting with a healthcare professional or registered dietitian before starting the keto diet is advisable to ensure it aligns with your health goals and needs. Remember that successful weight loss involves a holistic approach, including diet, exercise, and lifestyle choices.

2.6 Mediterranean Diet

The Mediterranean diet is often hailed as one of the healthiest diets in the world, and it has gained popularity not only for its potential health benefits but also for its effectiveness in promoting weight loss. This dietary pattern is inspired by the traditional eating habits of people living in countries bordering the Mediterranean Sea, such as Greece, Italy, and Spain. It's characterized by a balanced and diverse range of foods that provide numerous nutrients and can support weight management. In this comprehensive explanation, we'll explore the foods involved in the Mediterranean diet, its potential benefits for weight loss, and essential considerations for those looking to adopt this lifestyle.

Foods Involved in the Mediterranean Diet for Weight Loss:

1. Abundant Plant-Based Foods:
   - Fruits and Vegetables: Fresh, seasonal produce is a staple, providing essential vitamins, minerals, and fiber.
   - Legumes: Beans, lentils, and chickpeas are rich in fiber and protein, promoting satiety.
   - Whole Grains: Foods like whole wheat bread, bulgur, and quinoa

provide sustained energy and fiber.

2. Healthy Fats:
   - Olive Oil: Extra virgin olive oil is a primary source of healthy monounsaturated fats and antioxidants.
   - Nuts: Almonds, walnuts, and pistachios are consumed in moderation for their healthy fats and protein.
   - Seeds: Flaxseeds and chia seeds are nutrient-dense additions to meals.

3. Lean Protein:
   - Fish: Fatty fish like salmon and sardines are rich in omega-3 fatty acids.
   - Poultry: Chicken and turkey are lean protein sources.
   - Legumes: As mentioned earlier, legumes provide plant-based protein.

- Dairy: Greek yogurt and cheese are consumed in moderation.

4. Herbs and Spices: The Mediterranean diet emphasizes using herbs and spices like basil, oregano, and garlic for flavor, reducing the need for added salt.

5. Fruits for Dessert: Instead of traditional desserts, the Mediterranean diet often incorporates fresh fruit for a naturally sweet finish to a meal.

6. Wine in Moderation: Some people on the Mediterranean diet enjoy red wine in moderation, which may have cardiovascular benefits when consumed responsibly.

Potential Benefits of the Mediterranean Diet for Weight Loss:

1. Balanced and Sustainable: The Mediterranean diet is more sustainable

for many individuals because it doesn't involve strict restrictions, making it easier to maintain as a long-term lifestyle change.

2. Rich in Fiber: The diet is high in fiber from fruits, vegetables, and whole grains, which promotes feelings of fullness and can reduce overall calorie intake.

3. Healthy Fats: It includes healthy fats, such as those from olive oil and nuts, which can contribute to satiety and help control appetite.

4. Nutrient-Dense: The Mediterranean diet is rich in vitamins, minerals, and antioxidants, which support overall health and well-being.

5. Heart Health: This dietary pattern is associated with a reduced risk of heart disease, which is often linked to maintaining a healthy weight.

6. Weight Maintenance: While the primary focus of the Mediterranean diet is on overall health, many people find that it helps them maintain a healthy weight or lose weight when combined with portion control.

Important Considerations:

1. Portion Control: Even though the Mediterranean diet includes healthy foods, portion control is essential to ensure that calorie intake aligns with weight loss goals.

2. Physical Activity: Combining the Mediterranean diet with regular physical activity can enhance its effectiveness for weight management.

3. Individual Variability: Results may vary among individuals, and it's essential to listen to your body and make adjustments as needed.

4. Alcohol Consumption: If consuming alcohol, do so in moderation, and be aware of its calorie content.

5. Food Quality: The quality of ingredients is crucial. Choose high-quality olive oil and fresh, minimally processed foods for the best results.

In summary, the Mediterranean diet is a wholesome and balanced eating pattern that can support weight loss while providing numerous health benefits. Its focus on whole foods, healthy fats, and lean proteins, along with its flexibility, make it an attractive option for those seeking a sustainable and enjoyable way to manage their weight. As with any diet, it's important to personalize it to your individual needs and consult with a healthcare professional or registered dietitian for guidance if necessary.

Chapter 3: Exercise and Fitness

3.1 The Power of Cardiovascular Workouts

Cardiovascular workouts, often referred to as cardio exercises or aerobic activities, hold a special place in the realm of fitness and health. These workouts have long been recognized for their transformative power, offering a plethora of benefits that extend beyond just shedding pounds and building endurance. In this extensive exploration, we will delve into the world of cardiovascular workouts, understanding their significance, their impact on physical and mental health, and how they contribute to a better quality of life.

Defining Cardiovascular Workouts

workouts encompass a wide range of exercises that elevate your heart rate and increase your breathing rate for an extended period. These activities typically involve large muscle groups and are performed rhythmically. The primary goal of cardiovascular exercise is to enhance the efficiency of your heart, lungs, and circulatory system.

Types of Cardiovascular Workouts:

1. Running and Jogging: These high-impact exercises are excellent for improving cardiovascular fitness. They can be done outdoors or on a treadmill.

2. Cycling: Whether it's riding a bike outdoors or using a stationary bike, cycling provides an effective cardiovascular workout that's easy on the joints.

3. Swimming: Swimming engages various muscle groups and provides a full-body workout while being gentle on the joints.

4. Walking: Walking is a low-impact option that's accessible to almost everyone and can be easily incorporated into daily life.

5. Aerobics: Aerobic classes, such as step aerobics or dance aerobics, offer fun and social ways to get your heart rate up.

6. Jump Rope: A simple yet effective exercise, jumping rope can be done almost anywhere and is a fantastic calorie burner.

7. Elliptical Trainer: This machine simulates running or walking without the impact, making it suitable for individuals with joint issues.

8. Rowing: Rowing machines provide a full-body workout and are especially beneficial for building upper body strength.

9. HIIT (High-Intensity Interval Training): HIIT involves short bursts of intense exercise followed by brief periods of rest. It's time-efficient and can be done with various exercises.

10. Dancing: Whether it's Zumba, salsa, or hip-hop, dancing is not only a fantastic cardiovascular workout but also a great way to have fun.

The Transformative Power of Cardiovascular Workouts:

Physical Health Benefits:

1. Improved Cardiovascular Health: Cardio workouts strengthen the heart, enhance its pumping efficiency, and reduce the risk of heart disease.

2. Weight Management: Regular cardiovascular exercise burns calories, helping with weight loss or weight maintenance when combined with a balanced diet.

3. Enhanced Lung Function: Cardio workouts improve lung capacity and oxygen intake, which can boost overall stamina.

4. Lower Blood Pressure: Consistent aerobic activity can help lower blood pressure, reducing the risk of hypertension.

5. Better Cholesterol Profiles: Cardio exercises can raise HDL (good) cholesterol levels while lowering LDL (bad) cholesterol, promoting better lipid profiles.

6. Improved Blood Sugar Control: Regular cardio can help regulate blood

sugar levels, reducing the risk of type 2 diabetes and aiding in its management.

7. Enhanced Endurance: Cardiovascular workouts increase overall stamina and endurance, making daily tasks feel less strenuous.

Psychological and Mental Health Benefits:

1. Stress Reduction: Cardio exercises stimulate the release of endorphins, the body's natural mood elevators, which can help reduce stress and anxiety.

2. Better Sleep: Regular cardio workouts are associated with improved sleep quality and can help combat insomnia.

3. Increased Cognitive Function: Cardiovascular exercise has been linked to enhanced cognitive function, including improved memory and mental clarity.

4. Boosted Self-Esteem: Achieving fitness goals through cardio workouts can boost self-esteem and self-confidence.

5. Enhanced Mood: The release of endorphins during cardio can lead to a sense of well-being and positivity.

6. Reduced Risk of Depression: Cardiovascular exercise has shown promise in reducing the risk of depression and improving symptoms in those already diagnosed.

Longevity and Quality of Life:

Engaging in regular cardiovascular workouts is associated with increased longevity and a better quality of life. These exercises promote healthy aging by reducing the risk of chronic diseases and maintaining physical and mental function well into old age.

How to Incorporate Cardiovascular Workouts into Your Routine:

1. Set Realistic Goals: Start with achievable objectives, gradually increasing the intensity and duration of your workouts.

2. Find Activities You Enjoy: Choose activities that you find enjoyable to increase the likelihood of sticking with your routine.

3. Consistency is Key: Aim for at least 150 minutes of moderate-intensity cardio or 75 minutes of vigorous-intensity cardio per week, as recommended by health authorities.

4. Mix It Up: Vary your workouts to prevent boredom and overuse injuries.

5. Listen to Your Body: Pay attention to how your body responds to exercise, and don't push too hard too quickly to avoid injuries.

6. Warm-Up and Cool Down: Always start with a warm-up and end with a cool-down to prevent muscle strain and promote flexibility.

7. Consult a Professional: If you have underlying health concerns or are new to exercise, consult a healthcare provider or fitness professional before starting a new fitness regimen.

The power of cardiovascular workouts is undeniable, with their profound impact on physical health, mental well-being, and overall quality of life. Regular cardiovascular exercise can be a key factor in achieving and maintaining good health, helping you live a longer, more fulfilling life. Whether you're sprinting on a track, cycling through scenic routes, or dancing to your favorite tunes, cardiovascular workouts offer a pathway to a healthier, happier you. Embrace the transformative power of cardio, and let it propel you towards a life filled with vitality and well-being.

3.2 Strength Training and Muscle Building

Strength training and muscle building represent two fundamental aspects of physical fitness, with wide-ranging benefits that extend far beyond aesthetics. While many people associate these activities with bodybuilders or athletes, they hold immense value for individuals of all fitness levels and ages. In this comprehensive guide, we will explore the intricacies of strength training and muscle building, shedding light on their importance, the science behind them, and practical advice for incorporating them into your fitness journey.

Understanding Strength Training and Muscle Building:

Strength training is a form of exercise that focuses on improving muscular strength and endurance through resistance. This resistance can come from various sources, including free weights (such as dumbbells and barbells), machines, resistance bands, or even your body weight. The primary objective of strength training is to challenge your muscles, prompting them to adapt and become stronger.

Why Strength Training Matters:

1. Increased Muscle Mass: The most apparent benefit of strength training is muscle growth. As you repeatedly stress your muscles, they adapt by increasing in size and strength. This increased

muscle mass contributes to your body's functional abilities and can lead to improved athletic performance.

2. Enhanced Metabolism: Muscles are metabolically active tissues. The more muscle mass you have, the higher your resting metabolic rate (RMR). This means that even when you're at rest, your body burns more calories, which can aid in weight management and fat loss.

3. Improved Bone Health: Strength training places stress on your bones, stimulating them to become denser and stronger. This is especially important for preventing conditions like osteoporosis.

4. Better Joint Health: Strength training can enhance the stability and support provided by the muscles around your joints, reducing the risk of injury and promoting joint health.

5. Enhanced Functional Fitness: Strong muscles are essential for performing daily tasks with ease. Whether you're lifting groceries, carrying children, or simply navigating stairs, strength training can make these activities less physically taxing.

6. Injury Prevention: A well-balanced strength training program can address muscle imbalances and weaknesses, reducing the risk of injuries.

Muscle Building Science:

To understand muscle building, it's essential to grasp some fundamental physiological principles:

1. Muscle Hypertrophy: The process of muscle growth is called hypertrophy. It occurs when muscle fibers undergo stress and damage during exercise. In response to this stress, the body repairs

and reinforces the damaged fibers, leading to muscle growth.

2. Progressive Overload: To continue building muscle, you must continually challenge your muscles by increasing the resistance, repetitions, or intensity of your workouts. This principle, known as progressive overload, is the foundation of muscle building.

3. Nutrition Matters: Adequate protein intake is crucial for muscle growth. Protein provides the building blocks (amino acids) necessary for muscle repair and growth. Consuming enough calories is also essential to support muscle building, as an energy surplus is needed to fuel the process.

4. Rest and Recovery: Muscle growth doesn't occur during exercise but rather during the recovery phase. Getting sufficient rest, sleep, and proper

nutrition is essential to optimize muscle building.

Practical Tips for Effective Muscle Building:

1. Set Clear Goals: Define your muscle-building goals, whether it's increasing muscle size, strength, or endurance. Having specific objectives will help tailor your training program.

2. Resistance Training: Incorporate a variety of resistance exercises that target different muscle groups. Compound exercises (those involving multiple muscle groups) like squats, deadlifts, and bench presses are highly effective for muscle building.

3. Frequency: Aim for at least 2-3 strength training sessions per week, with a focus on targeting different muscle groups on different days.

4. Proper Form: Maintain correct exercise form to minimize the risk of injury and ensure that you're effectively targeting the intended muscles.

5. Nutrition: Consume a balanced diet that includes an adequate amount of protein to support muscle repair and growth. Consider consulting a registered dietitian for personalized guidance.

6. Rest and Recovery: Allow your muscles time to recover between workouts. Overtraining can hinder progress and increase the risk of injury.

7. Progression: Continually increase the intensity of your workouts by adding weight, increasing repetitions, or varying exercise variables.

8. Supplements: While not a substitute for a balanced diet, some individuals may benefit from certain supplements

like protein powder or creatine. Consult a healthcare professional before adding supplements to your routine.

Combining Cardio and Strength Training:

While strength training is pivotal for building muscle and increasing strength, cardiovascular exercise also plays a vital role in overall fitness. Combining both forms of exercise can help you achieve a well-rounded fitness profile, enhance cardiovascular health, and optimize calorie expenditure, which can be beneficial for weight management.

Strength training and muscle building represent essential components of a comprehensive fitness regimen. Their impact extends far beyond aesthetics, encompassing improved metabolic health, functional fitness, and overall well-being. By understanding the science behind muscle growth, adopting effective training strategies, and maintaining proper nutrition and recovery practices, you can harness the transformative power of strength training to achieve your fitness goals. Whether you're embarking on your muscle-building journey for the first time or seeking to refine your existing program, remember that consistency, patience, and dedication are key to realizing your full potential and reaping the numerous benefits of a strong, resilient body.

3.3 Yoga and Mindful Movement

Yoga and Mindful Movement for Weight Loss: A Holistic Approach

Weight loss is a multifaceted journey that goes beyond just diet and exercise. The integration of yoga and mindful movement offers a holistic approach to achieving and maintaining a healthy weight while fostering a deeper connection between mind and body. In this extensive guide, we will explore the profound impact of yoga and mindful movement on weight management, the science behind their effectiveness, and practical ways to incorporate them into your weight loss journey.

Understanding Yoga and Mindful Movement:

Yoga is an ancient practice originating in India that combines physical postures, breath control, meditation, and ethical principles. It emphasizes the union of mind, body, and spirit. Yoga comes in various forms, from gentle and restorative to dynamic and challenging.

Mindful movement encompasses a range of exercises that emphasize awareness, balance, and fluidity of movement. Examples include tai chi, qigong, Pilates, and mindful walking.

These practices focus on moving with intention and presence, promoting mental and physical well-being.

The Connection Between Mindfulness and Weight Loss:

Weight management often involves addressing not only the physical aspects of health but also the emotional and psychological components that influence eating habits and body image. Mindfulness, as a central element of yoga and mindful movement, plays a pivotal role in this process. Here's how:

1. Mindful Eating: Mindfulness encourages a heightened awareness of eating habits, helping you recognize physical hunger and fullness cues. It promotes slower, more deliberate eating, which can reduce overeating and emotional eating.

2. Stress Reduction: Mindfulness practices help manage stress, which is a common trigger for unhealthy eating habits. Reducing stress levels can lead to better weight control.

3. Emotional Resilience: Mindfulness fosters emotional resilience, enabling you to cope with negative emotions without turning to food for comfort.

4. Body Acceptance: Developing mindfulness can lead to greater body acceptance and reduced body dissatisfaction, which can positively influence weight loss efforts.

The Science Behind Yoga and Mindful Movement for Weight Loss:

1. Stress Hormones: Mindful practices like yoga can reduce the production of stress hormones such as cortisol. Elevated cortisol levels can contribute to

weight gain, particularly around the abdominal area.

2. Hormonal Balance: Yoga and mindful movement may positively affect hormones that regulate appetite and metabolism. For example, regular practice can improve insulin sensitivity and leptin levels, which play roles in hunger and satiety.

3. Reduced Inflammation: Chronic inflammation is linked to obesity and related health issues. Mindful practices have been shown to reduce inflammatory markers in the body.

4. Improved Sleep: Adequate sleep is essential for weight management. Yoga and mindfulness techniques can enhance sleep quality and duration.

5. Enhanced Self-Regulation: Mindfulness practices improve self-regulation skills, helping individuals

make healthier food choices and resist impulsive eating.

Practical Tips for Incorporating Yoga and Mindful Movement into Your Weight Loss Journey:

1. Start Slowly: If you're new to yoga or mindful movement, begin with beginner-friendly classes or routines. Gradually increase the intensity and duration as your fitness level improves.

2. Consistency is Key: Aim to practice yoga or mindful movement regularly. Even short sessions can be beneficial when practiced consistently.

3. Variety: Explore different forms of yoga (e.g., Hatha, Vinyasa, Restorative) and mindful movement practices to find what resonates with you.

4. Mindful Eating: Practice mindful eating by savoring each bite, chewing

slowly, and paying attention to your body's hunger and fullness cues.

5. Embrace Mindfulness Meditation: Incorporate mindfulness meditation into your daily routine. Start with short sessions and gradually increase the duration.

6. Breath Awareness: Focus on your breath during yoga and mindful movement exercises. Deep, conscious breathing can enhance mindfulness and reduce stress.

7. Professional Guidance: Consider attending classes led by certified instructors or working with a mindfulness coach or therapist to deepen your practice.

8. Holistic Lifestyle: Complement yoga and mindful movement with a balanced diet, regular exercise, and adequate

sleep for comprehensive weight management.

Yoga and mindful movement offer a unique and holistic approach to weight loss that addresses both the physical and emotional aspects of wellness. By incorporating mindfulness into your eating habits and physical activity, you can develop a deeper connection with your body, manage stress, and foster emotional resilience—all of which are essential for successful weight management.

Remember that the journey to weight loss is personal, and there's no one-size-fits-all approach. Yoga and mindful movement provide powerful tools to support your goals, but they are most effective when integrated into a well-rounded lifestyle that includes balanced nutrition, regular exercise, and self-compassion.

As you embark on this holistic journey toward weight loss, be patient with yourself and embrace the transformative power of mindfulness. With dedication and mindfulness, you can cultivate a healthier relationship with food, enhance your physical fitness, and achieve sustainable weight loss while nurturing your overall well-being.

3.4 HIIT (High-Intensity Interval Training)

High-Intensity Interval Training (HIIT) has emerged as a fitness phenomenon in recent years, offering a dynamic and efficient approach to weight loss. This revolutionary exercise strategy has captured the attention of fitness enthusiasts, athletes, and researchers alike due to its remarkable ability to burn calories, boost metabolism, and promote fat loss in a time-efficient manner. In this extensive guide, we will explore the science behind HIIT for weight loss, its numerous benefits, and practical tips for incorporating HIIT workouts into your fitness routine.

Demystifying High-Intensity Interval Training (HIIT):

HIIT is a form of cardiovascular exercise characterized by short bursts of intense activity followed by brief periods of rest or low-intensity recovery. The core principle behind HIIT is to challenge the body to work at its maximum capacity for short intervals, ultimately yielding substantial fitness and weight loss benefits.

The Science Behind HIIT for Weight Loss::

Caloric Burn: HIIT workouts demand high energy expenditure in a short time. During intense intervals, your body burns a significant number of calories.

This calorie burn continues even after your workout due to excess post-exercise oxygen consumption (EPOC) or the "afterburn" effect. EPOC requires additional energy to restore your body to its pre-exercise state, leading to additional calorie expenditure over time.

1. Metabolic Boost: HIIT can elevate your metabolism, enhancing your body's calorie-burning potential. This effect can persist for hours after your workout, aiding in weight loss efforts.

2. Fat Loss: HIIT has been shown to be particularly effective in reducing body fat, including visceral fat (the fat that surrounds internal organs). Visceral fat is associated with a higher risk of chronic diseases, making its reduction a crucial health goal.

3. Preservation of Lean Muscle Mass: Unlike some traditional steady-state

cardio workouts, HIIT helps preserve lean muscle mass while promoting fat loss. This is critical for maintaining a healthy metabolism.

4. Efficiency: HIIT offers time efficiency. You can achieve significant fitness gains and weight loss benefits in a shorter workout duration compared to longer, moderate-intensity exercises.

The Benefits of HIIT for Weight Loss:

1. Effective Fat Loss: HIIT promotes fat loss, particularly in stubborn areas like the abdomen and thighs.

2. Improved Cardiovascular Health: HIIT enhances cardiovascular fitness by improving heart health, lowering blood pressure, and increasing vascular function.

3. Enhanced Insulin Sensitivity: HIIT can improve insulin sensitivity, making it easier for your body to regulate blood sugar levels, which is vital for weight management.

4. Time Efficiency: HIIT workouts are shorter in duration, making it easier to fit into a busy schedule.

5. Variety: HIIT allows for a wide variety of exercises, preventing workout boredom and plateaus.

6. Applicability: HIIT can be adapted to various fitness levels and exercise preferences, whether you prefer running, cycling, bodyweight exercises, or strength training.

Practical Tips for Incorporating HIIT into Your Weight Loss Journey:

Consult a Healthcare Provider: Before beginning a new exercise program, especially HIIT, consult with a healthcare provider, especially if you have any underlying health conditions.

1. Start Slowly: If you're new to HIIT, begin with shorter intervals and lower intensity. Gradually increase the intensity and duration as your fitness improves.

2. Warm-Up and Cool-Down: Always start with a warm-up to prepare your body and finish with a cool-down to promote recovery and flexibility.

3. Interval Structure: HIIT intervals typically range from 20 seconds to 2 minutes, followed by equal or shorter rest periods. Experiment with different interval lengths to find what works best for you.

4. Frequency: Aim for 2-3 HIIT sessions per week, allowing adequate time for recovery between sessions.

5. Variation: Mix up your HIIT routines to keep workouts exciting and challenge different muscle groups.

6. Proper Form: Ensure proper exercise form to minimize the risk of injury. Consider working with a fitness professional or personal trainer if you're unsure about your form.

7. Hydration and Nutrition: Stay hydrated and maintain a balanced diet to support your HIIT workouts and overall health.

8. Listen to Your Body: Pay attention to your body's signals. If you experience pain, discomfort, or excessive fatigue, adjust your workout or take a rest day.

Sample HIIT Workout for Weight Loss:

- Jump Squats: 30 seconds
- Rest: 15 seconds
- Push-Ups: 30 seconds
- Rest: 15 seconds
- Burpees: 30 seconds
- Rest: 15 seconds
- Mountain Climbers: 30 seconds
- Rest: 15 seconds
- Repeat the circuit 3-4 times with a 1-2 minute rest between circuits.

High-Intensity Interval Training (HIIT) is a potent and time-efficient tool for weight loss that offers numerous physical and metabolic benefits. By incorporating HIIT into your fitness routine and complementing it with a balanced diet, you can achieve sustainable weight loss and improve your overall health.

Remember that the key to success with HIIT lies in consistency, progressive intensity, and listening to your body. As you embark on your HIIT journey, celebrate the transformative power of these high-intensity workouts and the remarkable impact they can have on your weight loss goals.

3.5 Dance and Fun Workouts

When it comes to weight loss, the idea of grueling workouts and strict diets may come to mind. However, achieving a healthier weight doesn't have to be dull or daunting. Dance and fun workouts offer a vibrant and enjoyable path to fitness that can make you forget you're even exercising. In this extensive guide, we'll explore the diverse world of dance and fun workouts, detailing various types, their benefits for weight loss, and practical tips to incorporate them into your fitness journey.

Types of Dance and Fun Workouts:

1. Zumba: Zumba is a high-energy dance workout that blends Latin and international music with choreographed dance moves. It's known for its lively atmosphere and calorie-burning potential.

2. Hip-Hop Dance: Hip-hop dance workouts incorporate popular hip-hop music and urban dance styles. They often focus on rhythmic and dynamic movements that engage the entire body.

3. Bollywood Dance: Bollywood dance workouts are inspired by the vibrant and expressive dance styles seen in Indian films. They combine traditional and contemporary moves, making for an exciting and calorie-burning experience.

4. Salsa: Salsa dancing is not only a romantic and energetic partner dance but also an excellent solo workout. It

involves fast footwork, spins, and body movements that provide a full-body workout.

5. Ballet Fitness: Ballet-inspired workouts, like Barre, incorporate ballet movements and techniques to strengthen muscles and improve balance.

6. Aerobics: Aerobic dance classes combine dance routines with traditional aerobic exercises to enhance cardiovascular fitness and burn calories.

7. Belly Dancing: Belly dance workouts focus on isolating and engaging various muscle groups, particularly the core. They promote flexibility, balance, and body awareness.

8. Hula Hooping: Hula hooping workouts involve spinning a hula hoop around your waist, hips, or arms. It's a

fun way to work on coordination and engage your core muscles.

9. African Dance: African dance workouts draw from the rich and diverse dance traditions of the African continent. They incorporate energetic and rhythmic movements that are both physically demanding and culturally enriching.

10. Pole Fitness: Pole fitness combines strength training, flexibility, and dance around a vertical pole. It's a unique and challenging workout that can help build upper body strength.

Benefits of Dance and Fun Workouts for Weight Loss:

1. Calorie Burn: Dance and fun workouts are highly effective for burning calories. The combination of movement, rhythm, and music can lead to substantial calorie expenditure.

2. Improved Cardiovascular Health: Dance workouts elevate heart rate and improve cardiovascular endurance, reducing the risk of heart diseases.

3. Enhanced Coordination and Balance: Dance workouts require coordination, balance, and agility, which can improve overall body control and prevent falls.

4. Increased Motivation: The enjoyment factor of dance and fun workouts can enhance motivation, making it more likely that you'll stick to your exercise routine.

5. Stress Reduction: Dancing and having fun while working out can reduce stress levels and improve mood, which can indirectly aid in weight management.

6. Social Interaction: Many dance classes provide a social environment that can foster connections and a sense

of community, making workouts more enjoyable.

7. Full-Body Engagement: Dance workouts engage various muscle groups, promoting overall body toning and muscle development.

Practical Tips for Incorporating Dance and Fun Workouts:

Choose What You Love: Select a dance or fun workout style that you genuinely enjoy. When you have fun, exercise becomes something to look forward to rather than a chore.

1. Start at Your Level: Don't be discouraged if you're a beginner. Most dance classes cater to all skill levels, so you can learn and progress at your own pace.

2. Set Realistic Goals: Define achievable fitness goals for yourself, whether it's

attending a certain number of classes per week, mastering specific dance moves, or losing a set amount of weight.

3. Consistency Matters: Consistency is key to seeing results. Aim for regular workouts, but also be flexible and forgiving with yourself on days when you can't exercise.

4. Mix and Match: Combine different dance and fun workouts to keep things interesting and prevent workout monotony.

5. Use Technology: There are numerous dance workout apps, videos, and online classes available, making it easier to incorporate dance and fun workouts into your daily routine.

6. Stay Hydrated: Dance workouts can be intense, so remember to stay hydrated and take short breaks as needed.

7. Dress Comfortably: Wear comfortable workout attire and supportive shoes appropriate for your chosen activity.

8. Consider Live Classes: Live dance classes, whether in-person or virtual, can provide real-time guidance and interaction with instructors and fellow participants.

9. Listen to Your Body: Pay attention to how your body feels during workouts. Rest and recover when necessary to avoid overtraining or injury.

Dance and fun workouts offer a joyful and engaging approach to weight loss and overall fitness. By embracing the rhythm,

3.6   Outdoor Activities and Adventure Sports

The quest for weight loss doesn't have to be limited to the confines of a gym or the monotony of indoor exercise routines. Outdoor activities and adventure sports present an exhilarating and natural path to achieving and maintaining a healthy weight. In this extensive guide, we'll explore the world of outdoor adventures and sports, the physical and mental benefits they offer, and practical ways to make them an integral part of your weight loss journey.

The World of Outdoor Activities and Adventure Sports:

Outdoor activities and adventure sports encompass a vast array of exhilarating pursuits, each offering unique challenges and rewards. Here are some popular options:

1. Hiking: Exploring scenic trails and natural landscapes on foot not only provides an excellent cardiovascular workout but also allows you to connect with nature.

2. Cycling: Whether on mountain trails or scenic roads, cycling is a low-impact activity that enhances leg strength and endurance while burning calories.

3. Running and Trail Running: Running outdoors offers fresh air and varied terrain, providing a more engaging and dynamic workout compared to treadmill running.

4. Swimming: Outdoor swimming, whether in lakes, rivers, or oceans, provides a full-body workout and is especially beneficial for individuals with joint issues.

5. Rock Climbing: Scaling natural rock formations or indoor climbing walls challenges your strength, balance, and problem-solving abilities.

6. Kayaking and Canoeing: Paddling through rivers, lakes, or coastal waters not only improves upper body strength but also offers a peaceful connection with water and nature.

7. Skiing and Snowboarding: Winter sports engage your core and lower body muscles while providing the thrill of gliding down slopes.

8. Surfing: Riding waves challenges your balance and strengthens your upper body, all while enjoying the beauty of the ocean.

9. Mountain Biking: Combining the joys of cycling with the excitement of rugged trails, mountain biking builds leg strength and endurance.

10. Adventure Races: These multisport events combine running, biking, paddling, and other challenges for a comprehensive fitness experience.

Physical and Mental Benefits of Outdoor Activities and Adventure Sports:

1. Calorie Burn: Many outdoor activities and adventure sports provide intense workouts that can burn a significant number of calories, aiding in weight loss.

2. Enhanced Cardiovascular Health: Engaging in outdoor physical activities can improve cardiovascular endurance, lower blood pressure, and reduce the risk of heart diseases.

3. Strength and Muscle Development: Activities like hiking, climbing, and kayaking engage various muscle groups,

promoting overall strength and muscle tone.

4. Mental Well-Being: Spending time in nature and participating in adventure sports can reduce stress, anxiety, and depression while boosting mood and mental clarity.

5. Improved Balance and Coordination: Outdoor activities often require balance and coordination, which can enhance overall physical fitness.

6. Natural Vitamin D: Exposure to sunlight during outdoor activities allows your body to produce vitamin D, which is essential for overall health.

7. Stress Reduction: The serenity of natural settings and the excitement of adventure sports can help you disconnect from daily stressors, promoting relaxation.

8. Sense of Achievement: Conquering physical challenges in outdoor environments can boost self-esteem and provide a sense of accomplishment.

Practical Tips for Incorporating Outdoor Activities and Adventure Sports:

1. Start Slowly: If you're new to outdoor activities or adventure sports, begin with beginner-friendly options and gradually progress to more challenging ones.

2. Safety First: Prioritize safety by wearing appropriate gear, staying hydrated, and adhering to safety guidelines and recommendations.

3. Learn Proper Technique: Consider taking lessons or seeking guidance from experienced individuals or instructors, especially for activities like climbing, skiing, or surfing.

4. Plan Ahead: Before heading out, plan your activities, know your route, check the weather, and inform someone about your plans.

5. Stay Hydrated and Nourished: Bring adequate water and snacks to fuel your adventures, especially during longer outings.

6. Warm-Up and Cool-Down: Begin with a warm-up and conclude with a cool-down to prevent injuries and muscle soreness.

7. Appropriate Footwear: Invest in quality footwear that suits your chosen activity to ensure comfort and reduce the risk of injury.

8. Mindful Exploration: Take the time to appreciate the natural beauty around you while engaging in outdoor activities. Mindfulness enhances the experience.

9. Join Groups or Clubs: Consider joining outdoor groups or clubs to meet like-minded individuals and gain new perspectives on outdoor fitness.

Sample Outdoor Adventure Day Plan:

1. Morning: Start with a hike or trail run in a nearby nature reserve, enjoying the serenity and fresh air.

2. Lunch: Have a picnic at a scenic spot, refueling with a balanced meal.

3. Afternoon: Try paddle boarding or kayaking on a nearby river or lake, engaging your core and upper body.

4. Evening: End the day with a relaxing yoga session outdoors, appreciating the tranquility of the setting.

Outdoor activities and adventure sports offer an invigorating and engaging approach to weight loss and overall well-being. By immersing yourself in the beauty of nature and embracing physical challenges, you can achieve your fitness goals while nurturing your mental and emotional health.

Remember that the joy of outdoor activities and adventure sports lies in the journey, not just the destination. Whether you're scaling a peak, gliding through water, or cycling along a scenic route, the sense of exhilaration and accomplishment is an integral part of the experience. So, lace up your hiking boots, grab your surfboard, or hop on your bike, and embark on an outdoor adventure that not only transforms your body but also enriches your soul.

Chapter 4: Lifestyle Modifications

4.1 Sleep and Weight Loss

In the pursuit of weight loss and overall health, many factors come into play, such as diet and exercise. However, one often underestimated and overlooked factor is sleep. Quality and quantity of sleep play a pivotal role in weight management, and understanding the complex interplay between sleep and weight loss is essential for anyone striving to shed pounds and lead a healthier life. In this comprehensive guide, we will delve into the profound impact of sleep on weight, the science behind it, and practical tips to improve your sleep and facilitate weight loss.

The Link Between Sleep and Weight:

The relationship between sleep and weight is intricate and multifaceted. Several key mechanisms underscore this connection:

1. Hormonal Regulation: Sleep has a profound influence on hormonal balance, particularly hormones that regulate appetite and metabolism.

2. Leptin: Leptin is a hormone that signals fullness and satiety. Inadequate sleep can lead to lower leptin levels, making you feel hungrier and less satisfied after meals.

3. Ghrelin: Ghrelin is a hormone that stimulates hunger. Sleep deprivation can increase ghrelin production, intensifying your appetite.

4. Insulin Sensitivity: Sleep plays a crucial role in improving insulin sensitivity. Poor sleep can lead to insulin resistance, making it more challenging

for your body to regulate blood sugar levels and increasing the risk of weight gain and type 2 diabetes.

5. Stress and Cortisol: Sleep is essential for managing stress, and chronic stress can lead to elevated cortisol levels. High cortisol levels can promote fat storage, particularly around the abdominal area.

6. Energy Balance: Sleep influences energy expenditure and calorie consumption. Fatigue resulting from poor sleep can lead to reduced physical activity and increased consumption of calorie-dense, high-carbohydrate foods.

The Science Behind Sleep and Weight:

1. Restorative Sleep: During deep, restorative sleep, your body undergoes crucial repair and recovery processes. This includes muscle and tissue repair, immune system support, and the

regulation of hormones involved in appetite control.

2. Sleep Cycles: Sleep is divided into cycles, including REM (rapid eye movement) and non-REM stages. These cycles influence memory consolidation, mood regulation, and metabolic processes. Interruptions in these cycles, often caused by sleep disorders or poor sleep quality, can disrupt these functions and affect weight regulation.

3. Circadian Rhythms: Your body operates on a circadian rhythm, a natural, internal process that regulates the sleep-wake cycle. Disruptions to this rhythm, such as irregular sleep patterns or exposure to artificial light at night, can lead to weight gain and metabolic disturbances.

Practical Tips for Improving Sleep and Supporting Weight Loss:

1.   Prioritize Sleep: Recognize the importance of sleep and prioritize it in your daily routine. Aim for 7-9 hours of quality sleep each night.

2. Establish a Routine: Sleep and wake up at the same time each day, even on weekends. This can help in regulating your body's internal clock.

3. Create a Sleep-Friendly Environment: Your bedroom should be conducive to sleep by keeping it dark, cool, and quiet. Consider using blackout curtains and white noise machines if necessary.

4. Limit Screen Time: Reduce exposure to screens (phones, tablets, computers, TVs) before bedtime, as the blue light emitted can interfere with your sleep-wake cycle.

5. Watch Your Diet: Avoid heavy meals, caffeine, and alcohol close to bedtime. These can disrupt sleep quality.

6. Stay Active: Engage in regular physical activity, but avoid vigorous exercise close to bedtime, as it can be stimulating.

7. Manage Stress: Incorporate stress-reduction techniques into your daily routine, such as mindfulness meditation, deep breathing exercises, or yoga.

8. Limit Naps: While short power naps can be refreshing, long or irregular napping during the day can interfere with nighttime sleep.

9. Limit Liquid Intake Before Bed: Minimize fluid intake in the hours leading up to bedtime to reduce the likelihood of waking up for bathroom trips during the night.

10. Seek Professional Help: If you have persistent sleep problems or suspect a

sleep disorder, consult a healthcare provider or sleep specialist for a diagnosis and treatment plan.

Sleep and Weight Loss Success Stories:

Case 1: Jane's Journey: Jane struggled with weight gain for years despite her efforts to diet and exercise. After improving her sleep habits and addressing her sleep apnea, she experienced a gradual but sustainable weight loss.

Case 2: John's Transformation: John, a busy professional, often sacrificed sleep to meet work demands. By reprioritizing sleep and implementing stress-reduction techniques, he not only lost weight but also saw improvements in his overall well-being.

Sleep is not merely a passive state but an active process that profoundly influences your weight and overall health. By recognizing the vital role sleep plays in hormonal regulation, metabolism, and energy balance, you can harness its power to support your weight loss journey.

Remember that sleep and weight loss are intrinsically linked, and neglecting one can hinder the success of the other. Prioritizing sleep, establishing healthy sleep habits, and seeking professional help when needed can be transformative steps on your path to a healthier weight and a more vibrant life.

4.2 Stress Reduction Techniques

In our fast-paced and demanding lives, stress is a near-constant companion. It not only affects our mental well-being but also plays a significant role in our physical health, particularly in the context of weight management. The intricate relationship between stress and

145

weight gain has been a subject of extensive research and exploration. In this comprehensive guide, we will delve deep into the complex interplay between stress and weight, the science behind it, and an extensive array of effective stress reduction techniques that can empower you on your weight loss journey.

Understanding the Stress-Weight Connection:

The connection between stress and weight gain is not as simple as a mere reaction to life's challenges. It is deeply rooted in the intricate interplay between our body's physiological responses and our emotional state. Here's a closer look at how stress can lead to weight gain:

1. Hormonal Havoc: Stress initiates a physiological response involving the release of hormones like cortisol and adrenaline. Cortisol, often referred to as the "stress hormone," plays a pivotal

role. Elevated cortisol levels, particularly in chronic stress, can lead to increased fat storage, predominantly in the abdominal area.

2. Appetite Altered: Stress has a significant influence on eating habits. For some, it triggers the desire for comfort foods, often high in sugar and fat, leading to overconsumption. Others may experience a loss of appetite or changes in food preferences.

3. Cravings Unleashed: Stress can provoke cravings, often for sugary and fatty foods. These cravings can become powerful drivers for overeating and weight gain.

4. Emotional Eating: Many individuals cope with stress by turning to food for emotional solace. Food serves as a source of comfort or distraction from stressors, resulting in emotional eating patterns.

5. Sleep Disrupted: Stress often disrupts sleep patterns, leading to sleep deprivation. The consequences of inadequate sleep can include hormonal imbalances that promote weight gain.

6. Exercise Evasion: The energy drain caused by stress can lead to reduced physical activity levels. When stressed, people may find it challenging to engage in regular exercise routines.

The Science Behind Stress and Weight Gain:

1. Cortisol's Role: Cortisol, the body's primary stress hormone, plays a pivotal role in the stress-weight connection. Chronic stress can lead to sustained elevated cortisol levels, which in turn can contribute to the accumulation of visceral fat, particularly around the organs in the abdominal cavity. This type of fat is linked to numerous health

issues, including insulin resistance and cardiovascular problems.

2.	Appetite's Tug-of-War: Stress disrupts the body's hunger and fullness cues. It can lead to overeating due to emotional factors or an inability to recognize true hunger. Moreover, stress can affect the brain's reward centers, making high-calorie foods more appealing and difficult to resist.

3. Blood Sugar Balancing Act: Stress influences blood sugar levels, potentially leading to cravings for sugary and starchy foods. These cravings, coupled with disrupted insulin regulation, can contribute to weight gain.

4. Metabolism Matters: Chronic stress can impact metabolic processes, potentially slowing down the metabolic rate. This change can make weight loss more challenging.

Effective Stress Reduction Techniques:

1. Mindfulness Meditation: Mindfulness involves focusing on the present moment without judgment. Regular mindfulness meditation can reduce stress levels and improve emotional regulation, ultimately aiding in weight management.

2. Deep Breathing Exercises: Practicing deep breathing exercises, such as diaphragmatic breathing or the 4-7-8 technique, can activate the body's relaxation response and reduce stress.

3. Progressive Muscle Relaxation: This technique involves systematically tensing and then relaxing different muscle groups, promoting physical and mental relaxation.

4. Yoga: Combining physical postures, breath control, and meditation, yoga is a

holistic practice that enhances flexibility, reduces stress, and supports weight management.

5. Tai Chi: This slow, flowing martial art focuses on balance and relaxation. Regular Tai Chi practice can reduce stress and improve overall well-being.

6. Biofeedback: Biofeedback techniques provide real-time data on physiological processes like heart rate and muscle tension. Learning to control these processes can help manage stress.

7. Journaling: Writing down your thoughts and feelings can be a cathartic way to process stressors and gain perspective on challenging situations.

8. Art and Creativity: Engaging in creative activities like painting, drawing, or crafting can be a therapeutic outlet for stress and a distraction from emotional eating.

9. Spending Time in Nature: Connecting with nature through activities like hiking or simply taking a leisurely walk in a park can provide a calming and grounding experience.

10. Social Support: Sharing your feelings and experiences with friends or a support group can provide emotional relief and help manage stress.

11. Limiting Caffeine and Alcohol: Reducing or eliminating caffeine and alcohol consumption, particularly in the evening, can improve sleep quality and reduce stress.

Case Studies: Success Stories of Stress Reduction and Weight Loss

Case 1: Sara's Transformation: Sara struggled with stress-induced emotional eating. Through regular mindfulness meditation and yoga practice, she learned to manage stress effectively, leading to significant weight loss.

Case 2: Mike's Journey to Wellness: Mike's high-stress job led to irregular eating habits and overconsumption of caffeine. By incorporating deep breathing exercises and biofeedback into his daily routine, he improved his stress management skills and successfully shed excess weight.

Stress is a ubiquitous part of modern life, and its impact on weight management should not be underestimated. Understanding the profound connections between stress, hormones, eating behaviors, and metabolism is crucial for anyone embarking on a weight loss journey.

By embracing effective stress reduction techniques, you can not only alleviate the emotional burden of stress but also create a supportive environment for sustainable weight loss. Remember that stress management is not a one-size-fits-all endeavor, and exploring different techniques can help you discover what works best for your unique needs and circumstances. Ultimately, the path to a healthier weight and a more balanced life begins with acknowledging the significance of stress reduction and taking proactive steps to manage it effectively.

4.3 Mindful Eating and Portion Control

In the quest for weight loss and improved health, it's not just what you eat that matters but also how you eat. Mindful eating and portion control are two powerful strategies that can help you achieve your weight loss goals while fostering a healthier relationship with food. In this extensive guide, we will delve into the principles and practices of mindful eating and portion control, exploring the science behind them, and providing practical tips to integrate them into your daily life.

Understanding the Significance of Mindful Eating and Portion Control:

Before delving into the details of mindful eating and portion control, let's first explore their significance in the context of weight management:

1. Mindful Eating: Mindful eating is about paying full attention to your food, savoring each bite, and being present in the moment during meals. It promotes awareness of your body's hunger and fullness cues, helping you make better food choices and avoid overeating.

2. Portion Control: Portion control involves managing the amount of food you eat, ensuring that you consume

appropriate serving sizes. It prevents excessive calorie intake, a common contributor to weight gain.

The Science Behind Mindful Eating and Portion Control:

Mindful Eating and Weight Loss:

1. Reduced Emotional Eating: Mindful eating can reduce emotional eating, helping you avoid consuming excess calories driven by stress, boredom, or other emotions.

2. Improved Food Choices: By paying attention to the sensory qualities of food (taste, texture, aroma), you're more likely to choose nourishing, whole foods over highly processed, calorie-dense options.

3. Enhanced Satiety: Mindful eating promotes better recognition of fullness

cues, preventing overeating and aiding in portion control.

Portion Control and Weight Management:

1. Calorie Control: Controlling portion sizes naturally limits calorie intake, which is essential for weight loss.

2. Regulated Hunger Hormones: Smaller, well-balanced portions can help regulate hunger hormones, reducing the likelihood of excessive snacking or overeating.

3. Psychological Satisfaction: Portion control can help satisfy psychological hunger without overindulging.

Practical Strategies for Mindful Eating and Portion Control:

Now, let's explore actionable steps to incorporate mindful eating and portion control into your daily routine:

1. Pause Before Eating: Take a moment before each meal to pause, breathe, and center yourself. This brief pause helps shift your focus to the act of eating and away from distractions.

2. Savor Each Bite: Pay attention to the flavors, textures, and aromas of your food. Engaging your senses enhances your eating experience and fosters mindful awareness.

3. Mindful Bites: Take smaller bites and chew your food slowly. This allows you to savor each mouthful and gives your body time to register fullness cues.

4. Listen to Your Body: Throughout your meal, check in with your body to assess hunger and fullness. Aim to stop eating

when you feel comfortably satisfied, not overly full.

5. Use Smaller Plates: Opt for smaller plates and bowls to help manage portion sizes. A smaller plate can create the illusion of a more substantial meal.

6. Pre-Portion Snacks: When snacking, avoid eating directly from a larger container. Instead, portion your snack into a small bowl or container to control intake.

7. Practice Mindful Shopping: Make a shopping list and stick to it. Avoid impulsive purchases of unhealthy snacks or larger quantities of food than you need.

8. Plan Balanced Meals: Create well-balanced meals that include lean proteins, whole grains, and plenty of vegetables. Balanced meals promote satiety and reduce the urge to overeat.

9. Hydrate Mindfully: Sometimes, thirst is mistaken for hunger. Stay hydrated throughout the day, and when you feel hungry, drink a glass of water before eating.

10. Mealtime Environment: Create a peaceful and enjoyable mealtime environment. Eliminate distractions like TV or smartphones, and set a pleasant atmosphere for dining.

11. Mindful Eating Journal: Keep a journal to record your eating experiences. Note your emotions, physical sensations, and any triggers for overeating.

12. Practice Gratitude: Take a moment to express gratitude for your food. Acknowledging the effort and resources that went into your meal can enhance appreciation and mindfulness.

Real-Life Success Stories:

Case 1: Lisa's Mindful Transformation: Lisa struggled with emotional eating and portion sizes. By practicing mindful eating, she learned to identify her emotional triggers and develop healthier coping mechanisms, leading to significant weight loss.

Case 2: John's Portion Control Journey: John used to consume large portions at each meal. By adopting portion control strategies and using smaller plates, he successfully reduced his calorie intake and achieved his weight loss goals.

Mindful eating and portion control are potent tools for weight loss and overall well-being. By cultivating awareness of your eating habits, recognizing hunger and fullness cues, and practicing portion control, you can develop a healthier relationship with food and take charge of your weight management journey. Remember that these practices require patience and consistency. Over time,

4.4 Habits and Behavioral Changes

In the journey towards a healthier, more fulfilling life, habits and behavioral changes stand as the cornerstones of lasting transformation. These small, everyday actions have the power to shape our well-being, influence our choices, and ultimately determine our path to success. In this in-depth exploration, we will delve into the fascinating world of habits and behavioral changes, uncover the science behind them, and provide practical insights on how to cultivate positive habits and sustain long-term transformation.

The Significance of Habits and Behavioral Changes:

Habits are the invisible architects of our lives. They are the routines, actions, and thought patterns that define how we interact with the world. Behavioral changes, in turn, are the conscious choices and actions we take to shift our habits in a more desirable direction. Here's why they matter:

1. Automatic Decision-Making: Habits, whether good or bad, often dictate our daily decisions with minimal conscious effort. By modifying these habits, we can shape our choices and behaviors in alignment with our goals.

2. Sustainability: Sustainable change is a gradual process, and habits are the vehicles that carry us toward our objectives over time. Developing positive habits ensures that we continue to progress even when motivation wanes.

3. Long-Term Impact: Transformative change isn't about quick fixes; it's about creating lasting improvements in our lives. Behavioral changes allow us to build a solid foundation for ongoing growth and development.

The Science Behind Habits and Behavioral Changes:

Understanding the mechanisms underlying habits and behavioral changes can empower us to make informed choices and optimize our efforts for personal transformation. Key aspects include:

1. The Habit Loop: At the core of every habit is a loop consisting of three elements: a cue (trigger), a routine (behavior), and a reward. Recognizing these components is essential for modifying or replacing habits.

2. Neuroplasticity: The brain's ability to reorganize itself by forming new neural connections is known as neuroplasticity. This phenomenon is pivotal in adopting new behaviors and altering existing ones.

3. Habit Stacking: Building on existing habits by adding new ones is a powerful strategy. It leverages the connections between established routines to create a seamless transition into new behaviors.

4. Self-Control and Willpower: Willpower is a finite resource. Understanding its limits and employing strategies to conserve and replenish it can aid in sustaining behavioral changes.

Cultivating Positive Habits and Behavioral Changes:

1. Set Clear Goals: Start by defining your objectives. What do you want to achieve

with your habits and behavioral changes? Having a clear vision provides motivation and direction.

2. Start Small: Begin with achievable, incremental changes. Overwhelming yourself with massive transformations can lead to burnout and discouragement.

3. Use SMART Goals: SMART goals are Specific, Measurable, Achievable, Relevant, and Time-bound. They provide a structured framework for setting and achieving objectives.

4. Understand Triggers: Identify the cues that prompt undesirable habits and the rewards associated with them. Knowing these triggers allows you to modify the habit loop.

5. Replace, Don't Eliminate: It's often more effective to replace a negative

habit with a positive one than to try to eliminate it altogether.

6. Practice Consistency: Consistency is the foundation of habit formation. Commit to practicing your desired behavior regularly, even on days when motivation is low.

7. Track Progress: Keeping a journal or using habit-tracking apps can help you monitor your progress and stay accountable.

8. Seek Social Support: Share your goals with friends, family, or a support group. Accountability and encouragement from others can be instrumental in maintaining positive changes.

9. Reward Yourself: Design a system of rewards for reaching milestones in your journey. Celebrating achievements reinforces the positive behaviors you're cultivating.

10. Mindfulness and Self-Awareness: Develop mindfulness practices to increase self-awareness. Mindfulness helps you recognize and manage the impulses and triggers that affect your habits.

11. Real-Life Success Stories: Transformations Through Habit and Behavioral Changes

Lena's Health Journey: Lena struggled with a sedentary lifestyle and unhealthy eating habits. By starting small and gradually incorporating daily walks and mindful meal planning, she lost weight and gained vitality over time.

Mark's Financial Makeover: Mark was drowning in debt due to impulsive spending. He initiated a habit of tracking his expenses daily and setting budgets. Over months and years, he cleared his debt and cultivated responsible spending habits.

Habits and behavioral changes are the foundation of personal growth and transformation. Whether your goal is to improve your physical health, enhance your financial well-being, or elevate your overall quality of life, understanding the science of habit formation and behavioral change is crucial.

By recognizing the power of small, consistent actions and adopting strategies for setting and achieving goals, you can embark on a journey of profound personal transformation. Remember that change is not an event but a process, and the habits you cultivate today have the potential to shape a brighter tomorrow. Embrace the journey, savor the progress, and relish in the life-altering potential of your habits and behavioral changes.

4.5 Support Systems and Accountability

Embarking on a weight loss journey can be a challenging endeavor, filled with ups and downs. However, you don't have to face this journey alone. Support systems and accountability play a pivotal role in achieving and sustaining weight loss success. In this extensive guide, we will delve into the profound impact of support systems and accountability on weight management, explore the science behind them, and provide practical strategies to harness their power for your benefit.

Understanding the Importance of Support Systems:

Support systems encompass a network of individuals, resources, and tools that provide encouragement, motivation, and assistance on your weight loss journey. They can include:

1. Friends and Family: Loved ones who offer emotional support, encouragement, and understanding as you work toward your weight loss goals.

2. Healthcare Professionals: Medical professionals, such as dietitians, nutritionists, and personal trainers, who can provide expert guidance and personalized plans.

3. Support Groups: Communities of individuals facing similar challenges, where you can share experiences, gain insights, and receive encouragement.

4. Online Communities: Virtual support networks through social media, forums, or weight loss apps, offering a sense of community and a platform for sharing progress.

5. Accountability Partners: A trusted individual who holds you responsible for your weight loss efforts, offering motivation and support.

The Science Behind Support Systems and Weight Loss:

1. Emotional Well-Being: Support systems provide emotional support, reducing stress, anxiety, and depression, which are common obstacles to successful weight loss.

2. Motivation and Commitment: Having people who believe in your goals and encourage your efforts can boost your motivation and commitment to weight loss.

3. Accountability: Support systems create accountability, making you more likely to adhere to your weight loss plan and resist temptations.

4. Knowledge and Guidance: Access to expert advice and resources within your support system can improve your understanding of nutrition, exercise, and healthy habits.

Accountability: The Backbone of Weight Loss Success:

Accountability refers to the practice of taking responsibility for your actions and being answerable to someone or something for your progress. In the context of weight loss, accountability can be a powerful catalyst for change. Here's why it matters:

1. Goal Setting: Accountability helps you set clear and realistic weight loss goals,

breaking them down into manageable steps.

2. Tracking Progress: Regularly monitoring your progress and sharing it with an accountability partner provides feedback and helps you stay on track.

3. Staying Committed: Knowing that you're answerable to someone or a group can motivate you to stick to your weight loss plan even when faced with challenges.

4. Problem Solving: When obstacles arise, accountability partners can offer insights and solutions, preventing you from feeling stuck.

5. Celebrating Success: Sharing your victories with someone who supports you can boost your confidence and reinforce positive behaviors.

Practical Strategies for Building Support Systems and Accountability:

1. Communicate Your Goals: Share your weight loss goals with friends, family, or a support group. Transparent communication can lead to increased understanding and support.

2. Seek Professional Guidance: Consult healthcare professionals, such as dietitians and personal trainers, for expert advice tailored to your needs.

3. Join a Support Group: Explore local or online support groups that align with your weight loss goals and preferences.

4. Use Technology: Utilize weight loss apps and online communities to track your progress and connect with like-minded individuals.

175

5. Find an Accountability Partner: Identify a trusted friend, family member, or colleague who can serve as your accountability partner. Set clear expectations and regular check-ins.

6. Create a Rewards System: Establish a rewards system to celebrate your achievements, both big and small, as a source of motivation.

7. Set SMART Goals: Make your weight loss goals Specific, Measurable, Achievable, Relevant, and Time-bound to facilitate tracking and accountability.

8. Regularly Assess Your Progress: Schedule regular assessments of your progress to identify areas for improvement and celebrate successes.

9. Join a Fitness Class or Group: Participating in group fitness classes or sports can provide built-in accountability and social support.

10. Real-Life Success Stories: The Impact of Support Systems and Accountability

Case 1: Emily's Journey: Emily struggled with yo-yo dieting for years. However, after joining a local weight loss support group, she found encouragement and motivation that led to sustainable weight loss.

Case 2: David's Transformation: David's busy work schedule often derailed his weight loss efforts. By enlisting his spouse as an accountability partner and scheduling regular check-ins, he stayed committed and achieved his goals.

The path to successful weight loss is not a solitary one. Building robust support systems and embracing accountability can be transformative steps on your journey. The emotional and motivational support provided by friends, family, healthcare professionals, and support groups can bolster your resilience and empower you to overcome challenges.

Remember that accountability is not about blame or judgment; it's about progress and growth. By creating a supportive environment and being answerable to yourself and others, you can unlock your full potential for weight loss success. So, reach out, connect, and share your goals with those who believe in your ability to achieve them, and together,

Chapter 5: Weight Loss Supplements and Tools

5.1 Understanding Supplements and Their Risks

In the ever-evolving world of weight loss, individuals often seek quick and easy solutions to shed excess pounds. Weight loss supplements have gained popularity as a convenient way to accelerate the process. However, understanding these supplements and their potential risks is crucial for informed and safe use. In this comprehensive guide, we will explore weight loss supplements, their mechanisms, the science behind them, and the potential risks associated with their consumption.

Weight Loss Supplements: An Overview

Weight loss supplements, often marketed as dietary supplements, come in various forms, including pills, capsules, powders, and liquids. They claim to aid weight loss by boosting metabolism, suppressing appetite, increasing energy expenditure, or blocking the absorption of fat. Common ingredients found in these supplements include:

1. Caffeine: A stimulant that can increase metabolism and reduce appetite temporarily.

2. Green Tea Extract: Contains antioxidants and compounds that may enhance fat oxidation and metabolism.

3. Garcinia Cambogia: Claims to inhibit fat production and reduce appetite.

4. Conjugated Linoleic Acid (CLA): Marketed as a fat-burning supplement that can reduce body fat.

5. Glucomannan: A fiber derived from the root of the konjac plant, it swells in the stomach to create a feeling of fullness.

6. Hydroxycitric Acid (HCA): Found in Garcinia Cambogia, it's marketed as a fat blocker and appetite suppressant.

7. Raspberry Ketones: Claimed to increase fat breakdown and metabolism.

8. Bitter Orange: Contains synephrine, which is marketed as a fat burner and appetite suppressant.

The Science Behind Weight Loss Supplements:

While some weight loss supplements have shown promise in laboratory studies or animal models, their effects in humans are often less conclusive. The science behind these supplements varies:

1. Caffeine: Caffeine is a well-studied stimulant that can temporarily increase metabolism and alertness. It may help burn more calories, but its effects tend to diminish over time as the body builds tolerance.

2. Green Tea Extract: Green tea contains compounds called catechins that have been linked to improved metabolism and fat oxidation. However, the amount of catechins in a typical supplement may not be sufficient to yield significant weight loss.

3. Garcinia Cambogia: Studies on Garcinia Cambogia have produced mixed results, with some suggesting modest weight loss effects, while others found no significant benefit.

4. CLA: Conjugated Linoleic Acid has shown some promise in reducing body fat in animal studies, but human trials have been inconclusive.

5. Glucomannan: Glucomannan, a water-soluble fiber, can increase feelings of fullness and reduce calorie intake when consumed with water. However, it is not a direct fat burner.

6. HCA: Hydroxycitric Acid in Garcinia Cambogia has not consistently demonstrated significant weight loss effects in human studies.

7. Raspberry Ketones: Limited research exists on raspberry ketones' effects in humans, and the available evidence is insufficient to support their weight loss claims.

8. Bitter Orange: Bitter orange contains synephrine, which may slightly increase

metabolism, but it has been associated with side effects and potential health risks.

Potential Risks and Concerns:

1. Safety: The safety of weight loss supplements varies widely. Some may contain hidden or harmful ingredients, and their long-term effects are often unknown.

2. Side Effects: Many weight loss supplements can cause side effects such as jitters, increased heart rate, digestive issues, and sleep disturbances.

3. Dependency: Some supplements with stimulants like caffeine can lead to dependency and withdrawal symptoms when discontinued.

4. Interactions: Weight loss supplements can interact with

medications or exacerbate pre-existing medical conditions.

5. Lack of Regulation: The dietary supplement industry is not as tightly regulated as pharmaceuticals, making it challenging to ensure the safety and efficacy of products.

6. Lack of Sustained Results: Even if weight loss occurs initially, supplements often fail to provide sustained results when not combined with diet and exercise changes.

7. Financial Cost: The cost of purchasing weight loss supplements can add up over time, with no guarantee of significant weight loss.

The Importance of a Balanced Approach:

Achieving and maintaining a healthy weight involves more than just taking supplements. A balanced approach includes:

1. Nutrition: Focus on a well-rounded, balanced diet rich in fruits, vegetables, lean proteins, whole grains, and healthy fats.

2. Physical Activity: Incorporate regular physical activity into your routine, combining aerobic exercises, strength training, and flexibility work.

3. Behavioral Changes: Address the root causes of overeating and unhealthy habits through behavioral changes, such as mindful eating and stress management.

4. Support and Accountability: Seek support from healthcare professionals, registered dietitians, or support groups to help you make sustainable changes.

5. Lifestyle Modifications: Make long-term lifestyle modifications that promote overall well-being, including improved sleep and stress management.

Weight loss supplements may promise quick solutions, but their efficacy and safety are often questionable. It's crucial to approach weight loss with a balanced, sustainable plan that includes a nutritious diet, regular physical activity, behavioral changes, and, if needed, guidance from healthcare professionals. Before considering any weight loss supplement, consult with a healthcare provider to assess potential risks and benefits in the context of your individual health and weight loss goals. Remember that achieving and maintaining a healthy weight is a journey that requires patience, commitment, and a comprehensive approach that prioritizes your overall well-being.

5.2 Wearable Fitness Technology

In the age of technological advancement, achieving weight loss goals has become more accessible, efficient, and engaging thanks to wearable fitness technology. These innovative devices, ranging from fitness trackers and smartwatches to heart rate monitors and smart clothing, have revolutionized the way we approach weight loss. In this comprehensive guide, we will explore the world of wearable fitness technology, delve into its mechanisms, investigate the science behind its effectiveness, and unveil practical strategies to harness its power for successful weight loss.

The Rise of Wearable Fitness Technology:

Wearable fitness technology refers to electronic devices and accessories designed to monitor and track various aspects of physical activity and health.

They have gained immense popularity in recent years due to their versatility and ability to provide real-time data. Key features of wearable fitness technology include:

1. Activity Tracking: Counting steps, monitoring distance traveled, and estimating calorie expenditure.

2. Heart Rate Monitoring: Tracking heart rate zones during exercise and rest for more accurate calorie burn calculations.

3. Sleep Tracking: Analyzing sleep patterns to assess sleep quality and duration.

4. GPS and Location Tracking: Monitoring routes during outdoor activities like running and cycling.

5. Smart Notifications: Receiving calls, messages, and app alerts directly on the device.

6. Health Metrics: Monitoring metrics such as blood pressure, blood oxygen levels, and body temperature in advanced devices.

7. Integration with Mobile Apps: Syncing data with smartphone apps for comprehensive health tracking.

The Science Behind Wearable Fitness Technology:

The effectiveness of wearable fitness technology in supporting weight loss is grounded in several scientific principles:

1. Motivation and Awareness: Wearable devices provide real-time feedback on activity levels, motivating users to move more and make healthier choices.

2. Goal Setting: Setting specific, measurable goals with wearable technology can enhance adherence to fitness and weight loss routines.

3. Accountability: Sharing progress and data with friends or social networks can create a sense of accountability, encouraging individuals to stay on track.

4. Data-Driven Decision-Making: Tracking metrics like calorie burn, heart rate, and sleep patterns enables individuals to make informed decisions about their fitness and nutrition.

5. Behavioral Psychology: Wearable devices employ principles of behavioral psychology, such as positive reinforcement and goal reinforcement, to promote healthier habits.

Practical Strategies for Harnessing Wearable Fitness Technology:

191

1. Choose the Right Device: Select a wearable device that aligns with your specific fitness and weight loss goals. Consider factors like the type of exercise you prefer, budget, and desired features.

2. Set Clear Goals: Establish specific, measurable, and time-bound goals using your wearable device. Whether it's daily step counts or weekly calorie burn targets, clear goals keep you motivated.

3. Monitor Progress Regularly: Consistently track your activity, sleep, and other relevant metrics. Review your data to identify patterns, set new goals, and make adjustments to your routines.

4. Stay Connected: Utilize the social features of your wearable device to connect with friends or participate in fitness challenges. Sharing achievements and progress can enhance motivation.

5. Integrate with Apps: Sync your wearable device with health and fitness apps to access a broader range of features, nutrition tracking, and personalized recommendations.

6. Personalize Your Workouts: Many wearables offer guided workouts and exercise routines. Tailor your workouts to your fitness level and preferences for maximum effectiveness.

7. Track Nutrition: Some wearables allow you to log your food intake. Combining activity tracking with nutrition monitoring can provide a holistic view of your weight loss journey.

8. Sleep Optimization: Pay attention to your sleep data to identify areas for improvement. Adjust your sleep routine to ensure restful, quality sleep, which is crucial for weight loss.

Real-Life Success Stories: The Impact of Wearable Fitness Technology

Case 1: Sarah's Transformation: Sarah struggled to stay motivated and consistent with her exercise routine. After incorporating a fitness tracker into her daily life, she saw significant improvements in her activity levels and lost weight steadily.

Case 2: Mark's Journey to Wellness: Mark had a sedentary lifestyle and was unaware of his activity levels. With a smartwatch that tracked his steps and provided reminders to move, he gradually increased his physical activity, leading to successful weight loss.

Wearable fitness technology is not merely a trend; it has become a valuable tool in the pursuit of weight loss and improved health. These devices empower individuals by providing data, motivation, and accountability, making it easier to set and achieve fitness goals.

Remember that wearable fitness technology is most effective when integrated into a comprehensive approach that includes balanced nutrition, regular exercise, and healthy lifestyle choices. By embracing this innovative technology, you can turn your weight loss journey into a dynamic and data-driven adventure, ultimately leading to a healthier, more vibrant life.

5.3 Meal Replacement Shakes and Bars

In the realm of weight loss and dieting, meal replacement shakes and bars have gained popularity as convenient options for those seeking to shed pounds. These products offer the promise of a quick and hassle-free approach to managing calorie intake. However, their effectiveness, nutritional value, and potential pros and cons are subjects of ongoing debate. In this extensive guide, we will explore meal replacement shakes and bars, their mechanisms, their place in weight loss strategies, and provide insights into their usage.

Understanding Meal Replacement Shakes and Bars:

Meal replacement shakes and bars are specially formulated products designed to serve as a substitute for one or more regular meals. They typically come in a variety of flavors and are available in pre-packaged, ready-to-drink form or as powders and bars that can be mixed or consumed on-the-go. The key components of these products usually include:

1. Proteins: Protein is a crucial component, often derived from sources like whey, soy, or plant-based proteins,

intended to help maintain muscle mass and provide a feeling of fullness.

2. Carbohydrates: Carbohydrates, primarily from sources like oats or fibers, provide energy and promote a sense of satiety.

3. Fats: Healthy fats, such as those from nuts or seeds, are included for overall nutrition and satiety.

4. Fiber: Fiber content is often elevated to support digestive health and increase feelings of fullness.

5. Vitamins and Minerals: These products are typically fortified with essential vitamins and minerals to compensate for nutrients lost when replacing whole meals.

The Mechanisms Behind Meal Replacements:

197

Meal replacement shakes and bars are designed to work through several mechanisms to facilitate weight loss:

1. Calorie Control: By offering a predetermined calorie content, these products help individuals manage their daily energy intake effectively.

2. Portion Control: The pre-portioned nature of meal replacements helps prevent overeating and promotes portion control.

3. Nutrient Balance: They aim to provide a balanced mix of macronutrients (proteins, carbohydrates, fats) and micronutrients (vitamins and minerals).

4. Satiety Promotion: The inclusion of protein, fiber, and healthy fats is intended to create a feeling of fullness and reduce overall food consumption.

5. Convenience: Meal replacements offer a convenient, grab-and-go option for busy individuals who may not have time to prepare a full meal.

Effectiveness of Meal Replacement Shakes and Bars in Weight Loss:

The effectiveness of meal replacement shakes and bars in weight loss can vary from person to person and depends on several factors:

1. Caloric Intake: Weight loss success often hinges on overall calorie intake. If meal replacements are used to replace high-calorie meals and result in a calorie deficit, they can lead to weight loss.

2. Adherence: Consistency and adherence to a meal replacement plan are critical. Skipping or substituting meal replacements inconsistently may not yield the desired results.

3.   Behavioral   Factors: Meal replacements can help individuals control their intake, but they may not address underlying emotional or behavioral eating patterns.

4. Long-Term Sustainability: Some people may struggle to maintain a meal replacement-based diet over the long term, leading to weight regain once they return to regular meals.

5. Nutritional Quality: The nutritional quality of the meal replacement product plays a significant role. Opt for options that are nutrient-dense and low in added sugars.

Potential Benefits of Meal Replacement Shakes and Bars:

1. Convenience: They offer a quick and convenient way to manage calorie intake, especially for those with busy schedules.

2. Portion Control: Pre-portioned servings help prevent overeating and encourage portion control.

3. Nutrient Fortification: Many meal replacement products are fortified with essential vitamins and minerals, providing a nutritional boost.

4. Satiety: The protein and fiber content in meal replacements can promote a sense of fullness and reduce snacking.

5. Structured Eating: Meal replacements provide structure and eliminate the need for meal planning, which can be helpful for some individuals.

Potential Drawbacks and Risks:

1. Sustainability: Depending solely on meal replacements may not be sustainable in the long term and can

lead to weight regain once regular meals are reintroduced.

2. Lack of Variety: A diet based on meal replacements can become monotonous and lacks the variety and enjoyment of whole foods.

3. Nutritional Gaps: While fortified, meal replacements may not provide the same range of nutrients as whole foods.

4. Expense: High-quality meal replacement products can be costly over time.

5. Dependency: Relying heavily on meal replacements may foster a dependency on these products rather than teaching healthy eating habits.

Using Meal Replacement Shakes and Bars Wisely:

If you choose to incorporate meal replacement shakes and bars into your weight loss strategy, consider these guidelines:

1. Consult a Healthcare Professional: Seek guidance from a healthcare provider or registered dietitian to ensure meal replacements align with your health and weight loss goals.

2. Diversify Your Diet: Use meal replacements as a supplement to a balanced diet rather than a complete replacement. Include a variety of whole foods for overall nutrition.

3. Behavioral Changes: Address emotional or behavioral eating patterns alongside the use of meal replacements for sustainable weight loss.

4. Regular Exercise: Combine meal replacements with regular physical activity for enhanced results.

5. Read Labels: Choose products with minimal added sugars, adequate protein, and a range of essential nutrients.

6. Stay Hydrated: Ensure you drink plenty of water when consuming meal replacements, as they can be dehydrating.

7. Monitor Progress: Keep track of your progress and adjust your plan as needed with the guidance of a healthcare professional.

Meal replacement shakes and bars can be effective tools in a weight loss strategy when used mindfully and as part of a holistic approach. They offer convenience, portion control, and nutritional benefits. However, it's essential to recognize their limitations and consider factors like long-term sustainability and adherence.

For sustainable weight loss and overall health, meal replacements should complement a balanced diet rich in whole foods and be part of a broader plan that includes behavior modification, regular exercise, and the guidance of healthcare professionals. Ultimately, the key to successful weight loss is finding an approach that aligns with your individual needs, preferences, and lifestyle.

5.4 Weight Loss Apps and Trackers

In today's tech-driven world, smartphones and wearable devices have become indispensable tools for managing various aspects of our lives, including health and fitness. Weight loss apps and trackers have emerged as powerful allies for individuals striving to shed excess pounds and improve their overall well-being. In this comprehensive guide, we will explore the world of weight loss apps and trackers, their features, their role in facilitating weight management, and the science behind their effectiveness.

The Rise of Weight Loss Apps and Trackers:

The prevalence of obesity and the pursuit of a healthier lifestyle have fueled the development of countless weight loss apps and trackers. These digital tools leverage the capabilities of smartphones and wearable devices to help individuals monitor their progress, make informed choices, and stay motivated on their weight loss journeys.

Key Features of Weight Loss Apps and Trackers:

Weight loss apps and trackers offer a wide range of features designed to support users in their weight management efforts. Some of the common features include:

1. Calorie Tracking: Users can log their daily food intake, track calorie consumption, and gain insight into their nutritional choices.

2. Exercise Logging: These apps allow users to record their physical activity, from workouts to daily steps, helping to gauge energy expenditure.

3. Goal Setting: Users can set specific weight loss goals, track progress, and receive reminders to stay on target.

4. Food Databases: Access to extensive food databases with nutritional information simplifies meal tracking.

5. Meal Planning: Users can plan balanced meals and create shopping lists to support healthy eating.

6. Community and Social Features: Many apps provide forums, social networks, and challenges to connect users and foster motivation and accountability.

7. Health Data Integration: Some apps sync with wearable fitness devices and collect data like heart rate, sleep patterns, and activity levels for a more comprehensive view of health.

The Science Behind Weight Loss Apps and Trackers:

The effectiveness of weight loss apps and trackers is grounded in established principles of behavior change and self-monitoring:

1. Self-Awareness: Self-monitoring, a central component of these tools, encourages users to become more aware

of their eating habits, physical activity levels, and progress toward their goals.

2. Goal Setting: Setting specific, achievable goals is a powerful motivator. These apps facilitate goal setting and provide ongoing feedback to track progress.

3. Accountability: Many apps promote accountability through features like food logging, which makes individuals more conscious of their dietary choices.

4. Motivation: Social features, such as connecting with others on similar journeys or participating in challenges, can boost motivation and adherence.

5. Feedback Loops: Real-time feedback on daily activities and goal attainment helps users adjust their behaviors for better outcomes.

6. Education: Nutritional information and meal planning tools can enhance users' understanding of healthy eating choices.

Benefits of Weight Loss Apps and Trackers:

1. Convenience: These digital tools offer convenience, enabling users to track their progress, log meals, and access information at their fingertips.

2. Awareness: Self-monitoring promotes self-awareness, helping users identify eating patterns, triggers, and areas for improvement.

3. Accountability: Logging meals and exercise routines fosters accountability, making it less likely for users to stray from their goals.

4. Motivation: The gamification elements and social features in many

apps can provide motivation and support.

5. Goal Attainment: Setting and tracking specific goals increases the likelihood of achieving them.

6. Data-Driven Decision-Making: Access to data and insights enables users to make informed choices about their health.

Potential Challenges and Considerations:

While weight loss apps and trackers offer numerous benefits, several challenges and considerations should be acknowledged:

1. User Engagement: Sustaining long-term engagement with these tools can be challenging, as user motivation may wane over time.

2. Data Accuracy: Users may encounter inaccuracies in food databases or discrepancies in calorie estimation, affecting the reliability of tracking.

3. Privacy and Data Security: Users should be cautious about sharing personal health data and ensure they are using reputable apps that prioritize data security.

4. App Overload: The plethora of available apps can be overwhelming. Users should choose apps that align with their goals and preferences.

5. Behavioral Change: While apps can provide valuable support, they do not replace the need for behavioral changes related to diet and physical activity.

Effectiveness of Weight Loss Apps and Trackers:

The effectiveness of these tools can vary widely depending on individual adherence, engagement, and the appropriateness of the chosen app for one's needs. Research has shown mixed results regarding the impact of weight loss apps on actual weight loss. Success is often contingent on the integration of app use with other lifestyle modifications, such as dietary changes and increased physical activity.

Choosing the Right Weight Loss App or Tracker:

Selecting the most suitable weight loss app or tracker is crucial for achieving positive outcomes. Consider the following factors when choosing an app:

1. User-Friendliness: The app should be easy to navigate and tailored to your preferences.

2. Compatibility: Ensure the app is compatible with your smartphone or wearable device.

3. Features: Select an app that aligns with your specific goals, whether it's calorie tracking, meal planning, or exercise logging.

4. Community and Support: Evaluate whether the app offers community features that can provide motivation and accountability.

5. Data Security: Check the app's data security and privacy policies to safeguard your personal information.

6. Reviews and Ratings: Read user reviews and ratings to gauge the app's effectiveness and user satisfaction.

7. Cost: Consider whether the app is free or requires a subscription, and assess its value relative to your goals.

Weight loss apps and trackers have revolutionized the way individuals approach weight management. These digital tools offer convenience, awareness, motivation, and accountability, making them valuable assets in the journey to a healthier you. While their effectiveness may vary, when used mindfully and in conjunction with other healthy lifestyle changes, weight loss apps and trackers can be powerful allies on your path to achieving and maintaining a healthier weight and overall well-being.

Chapter 6: Medical and Surgical Approaches

6.1 Bariatric Surgery Options

Obesity is a complex health concern that affects millions of people worldwide, with far-reaching implications for physical and emotional well-being. For individuals struggling with severe obesity, bariatric surgery can offer a life-changing solution. In this extensive guide, we will delve deep into the world of bariatric surgery, exploring the different surgical options available, their mechanisms, benefits, risks, and the life-altering impact they can have on weight loss and overall health.

Understanding Severe Obesity:

Severe obesity, often defined as having a body mass index (BMI) of 40 or higher, or a BMI of 35 or higher with obesity-related comorbidities, can significantly impair an individual's quality of life and increase the risk of various health issues, including type 2 diabetes, heart disease, sleep apnea, and joint problems. For many, lifestyle modifications, dieting, and exercise alone may not provide sufficient and sustainable weight loss.

The Role of Bariatric Surgery:

Bariatric surgery, also known as weight loss surgery, is a medical intervention designed to help individuals with severe obesity achieve substantial and lasting weight loss. These procedures aim to reduce the size of the stomach, limit food intake, and sometimes alter digestion, ultimately leading to significant weight loss and health improvements.

Types of Bariatric Surgery:

There are several types of bariatric surgery procedures, each with its unique mechanism and approach to weight loss. The most common procedures include:

1. Roux-en-Y Gastric Bypass (RYGB):

    - Mechanism: RYGB divides the stomach into a small upper pouch and a larger lower pouch. The small intestine is rerouted to connect to both pouches.

    - Benefits: Significant weight loss, improved type 2 diabetes control, reduced appetite, and changes in gut hormones that contribute to metabolic improvements.

    - Risks: Nutrient deficiencies, dumping syndrome (nausea, vomiting, diarrhea), and potential long-term complications.

2. Sleeve Gastrectomy:

- Mechanism: Sleeve gastrectomy involves removing a significant portion of the stomach, leaving a smaller, banana-shaped pouch.

- Benefits: Significant weight loss, reduced appetite, improved blood sugar control, and no rerouting of the intestines.

- Risks: Potential for leaks, acid reflux, nutrient deficiencies, and long-term complications.

3. Adjustable Gastric Banding (Lap-Band):

- Mechanism: An inflatable band is placed around the upper part of the stomach, creating a small pouch and a narrow passage.

- Benefits: Adjustable, reversible, no cutting or stapling, and fewer nutrient concerns.

- Risks: Slower and potentially less effective weight loss, band-related complications, and adjustment needs.

4. Biliopancreatic Diversion with Duodenal Switch (BPD/DS):

- Mechanism: BPD/DS combines a sleeve gastrectomy with intestinal rerouting, leading to reduced calorie absorption.

- Benefits: Significant weight loss, excellent diabetes control, and substantial improvements in metabolic health.

- Risks: Higher risk of nutrient deficiencies, malabsorption, and potential complications.

5. Gastric Balloon:

- Mechanism: A deflated balloon is inserted into the stomach and inflated, occupying space and promoting a feeling of fullness.

- Benefits: Non-surgical, reversible, and temporary weight loss aid.

- Risks: Temporary nature, potential for discomfort, and limited weight loss compared to other procedures.

Benefits of Bariatric Surgery:

Bariatric surgery offers a multitude of benefits beyond weight loss, including:

1. Sustained Weight Loss: Bariatric surgery typically results in significant and sustained weight loss, often

exceeding what is achievable through non-surgical means.

2. Improved Health: Many individuals experience improvements in obesity-related comorbidities, such as type 2 diabetes, hypertension, sleep apnea, and joint problems.

3. Enhanced Quality of Life: Weight loss can lead to increased mobility, reduced pain, improved self-esteem, and a better overall quality of life.

4. Metabolic Changes: Some procedures have a profound impact on metabolic hormones, improving insulin sensitivity and reducing appetite.

5. Long-Term Success: Bariatric surgery has demonstrated long-term success in maintaining weight loss and health improvements for many individuals.

Risks and Considerations:

While bariatric surgery can be life-transforming, it is not without risks and considerations:

1. Surgical Risks: All surgeries carry inherent risks, including infection, bleeding, and complications related to anesthesia.

2. Nutrient Deficiencies: Some procedures can lead to nutrient deficiencies, requiring lifelong supplementation and monitoring.

3. Psychological Factors: Addressing underlying psychological factors, such as emotional eating and food addiction, is crucial for long-term success.

4. Lifestyle Changes: Bariatric surgery requires significant dietary and lifestyle changes to maximize benefits and minimize risks.

5. Commitment: Long-term success requires a lifelong commitment to follow-up care, dietary guidelines, and lifestyle modifications.

6. Cost: Bariatric surgery can be costly, and insurance coverage varies. Understanding financial implications is essential.

The Importance of Multidisciplinary Care:

Successful bariatric surgery outcomes depend on a multidisciplinary approach involving healthcare professionals such as bariatric surgeons, dietitians, psychologists, and physical therapists. These experts collaborate to assess eligibility, provide preoperative counseling, and offer postoperative support.

Is Bariatric Surgery Right for You?

Bariatric surgery is a highly individualized decision. Consider the following factors when determining if it's right for you:

1. BMI and Health Conditions: Evaluate your BMI and the presence of obesity-related health conditions.

2. Commitment: Assess your commitment to lifelong dietary and lifestyle changes.

3. Psychological Evaluation: Undergo a psychological evaluation to address potential emotional eating or mental health concerns.

4. Medical Evaluation: Consult with a bariatric surgeon to determine eligibility and discuss surgical options.

5. Insurance Coverage: Explore your insurance coverage and financial considerations.

Bariatric surgery is a transformative option for individuals with severe obesity, offering the potential for substantial weight loss, improved health, and enhanced quality of life. However, it is not a one-size-fits-all solution, and the decision to pursue surgery should be made carefully in consultation with healthcare professionals. Bariatric surgery is a powerful tool, but its success ultimately hinges on a lifelong commitment to dietary, lifestyle, and emotional well-being changes. When used wisely and in conjunction with a comprehensive care team, bariatric surgery can be a life-altering step towards achieving a healthier, more fulfilling life.

6.2 Prescription Medications for Weight Loss

Weight management is a complex and challenging journey, and for some individuals, diet and exercise alone may not provide the desired results. Prescription medications for weight loss have emerged as a valuable option for those struggling with obesity or overweight conditions. In this extensive guide, we will delve deep into the world of prescription weight loss medications, exploring the different medications available, their mechanisms, efficacy, safety, potential side effects, and their role in helping individuals achieve and maintain a healthier weight.

The Challenge of Obesity:

Obesity is a prevalent health issue with far-reaching consequences for physical and mental well-being. It is associated with an increased risk of chronic diseases such as type 2 diabetes, heart disease, hypertension, and certain types of cancer. Weight loss is often recommended as a primary intervention for managing obesity and its related health complications.

When Lifestyle Interventions Alone Aren't Enough:

While lifestyle modifications, including dietary changes and increased physical activity, are essential components of weight management, they may not always yield significant or sustainable results, especially for individuals with severe obesity. Prescription weight loss medications are designed to complement these lifestyle changes and provide additional support to help individuals achieve their weight loss goals.

Common Prescription Weight Loss Medications:

Several prescription medications are approved for weight loss in the United States. Some of the most widely used and studied include:

1. Orlistat (Alli, Xenical):

- Mechanism: Orlistat works by inhibiting the absorption of dietary fats in the intestines, leading to reduced calorie intake.

- Efficacy: Studies have shown modest weight loss with orlistat, primarily when combined with a reduced-calorie diet.

- Safety: Side effects include gastrointestinal symptoms (oily stools, flatulence), and it can affect fat-soluble vitamin absorption.

2. Phentermine-Topiramate (Qsymia):

- Mechanism: This combination medication works as an appetite suppressant (phentermine) and an antiepileptic drug (topiramate) that may affect food cravings.

- Efficacy: Phentermine-topiramate has been associated with significant weight loss in clinical trials.

- Safety: Common side effects include dry mouth, insomnia, and potential neurological side effects like cognitive impairment and mood changes.

3. Bupropion-Naltrexone (Contrave):

- Mechanism: Combining an antidepressant (bupropion) with an opioid receptor antagonist (naltrexone) helps control appetite and reduce food cravings.

- Efficacy: Clinical trials have shown modest weight loss with bupropion-naltrexone.

- Safety: Side effects include nausea, headache, and potential risks associated with bupropion use.

4. Liraglutide (Saxenda):

- Mechanism: Liraglutide is a glucagon-like peptide-1 (GLP-1) receptor agonist that regulates appetite and reduces food intake.

- Efficacy: Saxenda has been associated with significant weight loss in clinical trials.

- Safety: Common side effects include nausea, vomiting, and potential concerns about pancreatitis and thyroid tumors (though rare).

5. Phentermine (Adipex-P, Lomaira):

- Mechanism: Phentermine is an appetite suppressant that works by increasing the release of norepinephrine, reducing hunger signals to the brain.

- Efficacy: Phentermine has been used for decades and is associated with short-term weight loss.

- Safety: It may cause increased heart rate, blood pressure, and potential for addiction or abuse.

Effectiveness of Prescription Weight Loss Medications:

The effectiveness of prescription weight loss medications varies among individuals and is influenced by factors such as the specific medication used, adherence to prescribed guidelines, and the presence of obesity-related comorbidities. Generally, these medications are more effective when combined with dietary modifications, increased physical activity, and behavioral counseling.

Safety and Potential Side Effects:

Prescription weight loss medications are not without risks. While they can be effective tools for weight management, they may also present potential side effects, which can vary depending on the medication:

1. Gastrointestinal Symptoms: Some medications, like orlistat, can cause gastrointestinal discomfort, including diarrhea and oily stools.

2. Cardiovascular Effects: Certain weight loss medications may increase heart rate and blood pressure, which can be concerning for individuals with cardiovascular conditions.

3. Neurological and Psychological Effects: Medications like phentermine-topiramate and bupropion-naltrexone may have side effects related to mood, cognition, and sleep.

4. Metabolic Effects: There may be concerns about effects on glucose metabolism, such as those associated with liraglutide.

5. Safety for Specific Populations: Some medications may not be suitable for

individuals with certain medical conditions or who are pregnant or breastfeeding.

Considerations Before Using Prescription Weight Loss Medications:

Before considering prescription weight loss medications, individuals should:

1. Consult a Healthcare Provider: Speak with a healthcare provider who can assess your eligibility and discuss potential risks and benefits.

2. Evaluate Lifestyle Modifications: Ensure that you have attempted lifestyle modifications, including diet and exercise changes, before seeking prescription medication.

3. Understand Potential Side Effects: Be aware of potential side effects and their implications for your health.

4. Monitor Progress: Regularly monitor your progress and adhere to your healthcare provider's recommendations.

Prescription weight loss medications can be valuable tools for individuals struggling with obesity or overweight conditions, especially when combined with lifestyle modifications. However, their use should be approached with caution, under the guidance of a healthcare provider, and with a clear understanding of potential risks and benefits. Weight loss medications are not a one-size-fits-all solution, and their efficacy may vary among individuals. A comprehensive approach to weight management, including dietary changes, increased physical activity, and behavioral counseling, remains essential for long-term success in achieving and maintaining a healthier weight and overall well-being.

6.3 Liposuction and Cosmetic Procedures

The pursuit of a healthier and more attractive body is a common aspiration for many individuals. While diet and exercise are fundamental to achieving these goals, there are situations where stubborn fat deposits and cosmetic concerns persist despite one's best efforts. In such cases, liposuction and other cosmetic procedures can offer transformative solutions. In this comprehensive guide, we will explore the world of liposuction and various cosmetic procedures for weight loss and body contouring, including their mechanisms, benefits, potential risks, and the role they play in enhancing both physical appearance and self-esteem.

Understanding Cosmetic Procedures for Weight Loss and Body Contouring:

Cosmetic procedures for weight loss and body contouring encompass a wide range of surgical and non-surgical interventions designed to improve one's physical appearance. These procedures can address concerns such as excess fat, loose skin, cellulite, and body proportions, ultimately enhancing body aesthetics and self-confidence.

Liposuction: Sculpting the Body Silhouette:

Liposuction, also known as lipoplasty or body contouring surgery, is one of the most common and effective cosmetic procedures for removing localized fat deposits. Here's an overview of liposuction:

- Mechanism: Liposuction involves the surgical removal of fat deposits from specific areas of the body through a cannula (a thin tube) and suction.

- Benefits: Liposuction can provide significant and immediate reduction in fat volume, improving body contours and proportions.

- Areas Treated: Common treatment areas include the abdomen, thighs, hips, buttocks, arms, and neck.

- Results: While results are visible soon after surgery, the full outcome may take several months to become apparent as swelling subsides.

Tummy Tuck (Abdominoplasty): Achieving a Flatter Stomach:

- A tummy tuck, or abdominoplasty, is a surgical procedure primarily focused on improving the appearance of the abdomen:

- Mechanism: Excess skin and fat are removed from the abdominal area, and weakened or separated abdominal muscles are tightened.

- Benefits: Abdominoplasty can create a flatter, firmer abdominal contour, particularly useful for individuals with loose skin and muscle laxity after weight loss or pregnancy.

- Recovery: Recovery time varies but typically includes a period of restricted activity and garment use for support.

Body Lift: Comprehensive Body Contouring:

A body lift, also known as a belt lipectomy, is a surgical procedure that addresses multiple areas of the body simultaneously:

- Mechanism: A circumferential incision is made around the lower torso, allowing for the removal of excess skin and fat from the abdomen, buttocks, and thighs.

- Benefits: Body lifts provide comprehensive body contouring and can dramatically improve the overall body silhouette.

- Candidates: Suitable for individuals with significant skin laxity and fat deposits, often following massive weight loss.

Non-Surgical Options: Minimally Invasive Techniques:

Non-surgical cosmetic procedures have also gained popularity for individuals seeking aesthetic improvements without surgery:

1. CoolSculpting: This non-invasive procedure freezes and destroys fat cells in targeted areas, which are gradually eliminated by the body's natural processes.

2. Laser Lipolysis (Laser-Assisted Liposuction): Laser energy is used to liquefy fat cells before suction removal, potentially reducing swelling and bruising.

3. Radiofrequency Skin Tightening: Radiofrequency technology tightens loose skin by stimulating collagen production, often used in conjunction with fat reduction procedures.

4. Cellulite Treatments: Various treatments, such as Endermologie and acoustic wave therapy, aim to reduce the appearance of cellulite by improving skin texture and elasticity.

Benefits of Cosmetic Procedures for Weight Loss and Body Contouring:

1. Enhanced Aesthetics: These procedures can lead to a more sculpted and attractive physique.

2. Improved Self-Confidence: Many individuals experience increased self-esteem and body confidence following successful cosmetic interventions.

3. Localized Fat Reduction: Liposuction and related procedures can target

specific problem areas that may not respond to diet and exercise.

4. Skin Tightening: Surgical procedures like tummy tucks and body lifts can address skin laxity, a common concern after weight loss.

5. Comprehensive Results: Body lifts offer all-encompassing contouring, addressing multiple areas in a single surgery.

Risks and Considerations:

1. Surgical Risks: All surgical procedures carry risks such as infection, bleeding, scarring, and anesthesia-related complications.

2. Recovery Time: Surgical procedures typically require a recovery period with post-operative restrictions on physical activity.

3. Results and Expectations: Realistic expectations are crucial, as outcomes may not always meet idealized goals.

4. Scarring: Surgical procedures leave scars, which vary in visibility depending on factors like incision placement and individual healing.

5. Cost: Cosmetic procedures are often elective and may not be covered by insurance, necessitating consideration of cost.

Choosing the Right Cosmetic Procedure:

Selecting the most suitable cosmetic procedure involves careful consideration of personal goals, body type, medical history, and consultation with a board-certified plastic surgeon or dermatologist. A comprehensive evaluation and discussion of options are essential to ensure that the chosen procedure aligns with individual needs and expectations.

Liposuction and cosmetic procedures for weight loss and body contouring offer transformative opportunities for individuals seeking aesthetic improvements. Whether through surgical interventions like liposuction, tummy tucks, or body lifts, or non-surgical approaches such as CoolSculpting and laser lipolysis, these procedures can provide enhanced body aesthetics and bolster self-confidence. However, it's vital to approach such interventions with a clear understanding of the potential benefits, risks, and commitment to post-operative care and recovery. Ultimately, the decision to pursue cosmetic procedures should be made in consultation with a qualified healthcare professional and aligned with one's personal goals and aspirations for physical transformation.

6.4   The   Role   of   Medical Professionals

In the battle against obesity and the pursuit of a healthier life, medical professionals play an indispensable role. Their expertise, guidance, and support are instrumental in helping individuals achieve and maintain weight loss goals. In this extensive guide, we will delve deep into the multifaceted role of medical professionals in weight loss, exploring their contributions across various healthcare disciplines, the importance of personalized care, and the evolving landscape of obesity treatment.

Understanding the Weight Epidemic:

Obesity, characterized by excess body fat, has reached epidemic proportions globally, with substantial implications for public health. It is associated with a myriad of health concerns, including heart disease, type 2 diabetes, hypertension, and certain types of cancer. While lifestyle factors such as poor diet and sedentary behavior contribute significantly to obesity, its management often requires a comprehensive healthcare approach.

1. The Multidisciplinary Team: Medical professionals in weight loss often work as part of a multidisciplinary team, collaborating to address the various aspects of obesity treatment. This team may include:

2. Primary Care Physicians (PCPs): PCPs serve as the initial point of contact for patients and play a critical role in assessing overall health, identifying obesity-related comorbidities, and referring patients to specialists as needed.

3. Dietitians and Nutritionists: Nutrition experts provide guidance on dietary modifications, meal planning, and calorie management tailored to individual needs and health goals.

4. Exercise Physiologists and Physical Therapists: These professionals design and supervise exercise programs, promoting physical activity as a key component of weight loss and overall well-being.

5. Endocrinologists: Specialists in hormonal disorders can help identify and manage underlying hormonal factors contributing to obesity.

6. Psychologists and Psychiatrists: Mental health professionals address emotional and psychological aspects of weight management, such as emotional eating, body image concerns, and mood disorders.

7.   Bariatric   Surgeons: Surgeons specializing in weight loss procedures like   gastric   bypass   and   sleeve gastrectomy offer surgical interventions for severe obesity.

8. Nurse Practitioners and Physician Assistants: These healthcare providers collaborate with physicians, offering primary care services and patient education.

The Role of Medical Professionals:

Medical professionals contribute to weight loss efforts in several key ways:

1. Assessment and Diagnosis: They assess patients' weight, overall health, and obesity-related comorbidities to establish a baseline and identify contributing factors.

2. Personalized Treatment Plans: Medical professionals develop individualized treatment plans that consider a patient's unique needs, medical history, and goals.

3. Education and Counseling: They educate patients about the principles of a balanced diet, physical activity, and behavior modification techniques necessary for sustainable weight loss.

4. Behavioral Support: Medical professionals address psychological and behavioral aspects of obesity, helping patients identify triggers for overeating and develop coping strategies.

5. Medical Interventions: In some cases, medical professionals may prescribe medications for weight management or recommend surgical interventions when appropriate.

6. Monitoring and Follow-Up: Ongoing monitoring and follow-up appointments allow healthcare providers to track progress, adjust treatment plans, and provide ongoing support.

7. Motivation and Accountability: Medical professionals offer motivation and accountability, empowering patients to stay on track with their weight loss journey.

The Importance of Personalized Care:

Personalization is a cornerstone of effective weight loss management. Medical professionals recognize that each individual's journey is unique, and there is no one-size-fits-all approach. Personalized care involves tailoring treatment plans to address not only physical health but also psychological, emotional, and social factors that influence weight.

The Evolving Landscape of Obesity Treatment:

The field of obesity treatment continues to evolve, with medical professionals at the forefront of research and innovation. Some noteworthy developments include:

1. Precision Medicine: Advancements in genetics and personalized medicine are shedding light on how an individual's genetic makeup can influence weight and metabolism, leading to more targeted treatment approaches.

2. Pharmacotherapy: Ongoing research is uncovering new medications and treatment strategies for obesity, expanding the toolkit available to medical professionals.

3. Behavioral Therapies: Innovative behavioral interventions, such as cognitive-behavioral therapy and

mindfulness-based techniques, are being integrated into obesity treatment plans.

4. Telehealth: The adoption of telehealth has made it easier for medical professionals to reach and support patients remotely, improving access to care, particularly in underserved areas.

5. Bariatric Surgery Advances: Surgical techniques for weight loss are continually evolving, with minimally invasive procedures and improved outcomes.

Challenges and Considerations:

While medical professionals play a crucial role in weight loss, several challenges and considerations are essential to acknowledge:

1. Stigma and Bias: Healthcare professionals must confront weight bias

and stigma, ensuring that all patients receive respectful and equitable care.

2. Long-Term Engagement: Sustaining patient engagement and adherence to treatment plans over the long term can be challenging.

3. Access to Care: Disparities in access to obesity treatment options, including surgical interventions, need to be addressed to ensure equitable care.

4. Interdisciplinary Collaboration: Effective teamwork and communication among healthcare disciplines are vital for comprehensive obesity care.

Medical professionals are instrumental in the battle against obesity, guiding individuals towards healthier lives. Their role extends beyond mere weight loss to encompass holistic well-being, addressing the physical, psychological, and emotional aspects of health. As the field of obesity treatment continues to evolve, medical professionals will remain at the forefront, offering innovative solutions, personalized care, and unwavering support to individuals striving to achieve and maintain a healthier weight and a better quality of life. Their contributions are essential in reshaping the narrative around obesity from one of stigma and despair to one of hope, empowerment, and lasting change.

Chapter 7: Mind-Body Connection

7.1 Mindful Eating and Intuitive Eating

In a world marked by hectic schedules, fast-food culture, and diet fads, the principles of mindful eating and intuitive eating offer a refreshing and sustainable approach to nourishing the body and soul. These practices transcend mere diets; they invite individuals to cultivate a mindful relationship with food, honor their bodies' signals, and develop a profound sense of self-compassion. In this extensive guide, we will explore the transformative power of mindful eating and intuitive eating, their origins, principles, benefits, and how they can reshape your approach to food and well-being.

Understanding Mindful Eating:

Mindful eating is a practice rooted in mindfulness, an ancient Buddhist meditation technique that involves paying attention to the present moment without judgment. In the context of eating, mindfulness encourages a heightened awareness of the sensory experience of food, the emotions surrounding eating, and the body's hunger and fullness cues.

Principles of Mindful Eating:

1. Present Moment Awareness: Mindful eating invites you to savor each bite by being fully present during meals. It involves engaging all your senses to appreciate the flavors, textures, and aromas of your food.

2. Non-Judgmental Observation: There is no room for guilt, shame, or criticism

in mindful eating. It encourages an open and non-judgmental awareness of your thoughts and feelings about food.

3. Listening to Hunger and Fullness: Mindful eating encourages you to tune in to your body's cues for hunger and fullness, helping you eat when you're genuinely hungry and stop when you're satisfied.

4. Satisfaction Over Quantity: Instead of focusing solely on portion sizes or calorie counts, mindful eating prioritizes the quality of your eating experience and the satisfaction derived from each meal.

5. Awareness of Emotional Eating: Mindfulness enables you to identify emotional eating behaviors and create healthy coping mechanisms for stress and negative emotions.

Benefits of Mindful Eating:

1. Improved Digestion: Being present during meals can enhance the body's digestive processes, reducing issues like bloating and indigestion.

2. Healthy Weight Management: Mindful eating promotes a balanced approach to eating, which can support both weight loss and weight maintenance.

3. Enhanced Enjoyment of Food: By fully savoring each bite, you can derive greater satisfaction from your meals.

4. Emotional Well-Being: Mindful eating promotes a healthier relationship with food, which can help lower stress, anxiety, and emotional overeating.

5. Increased Self-Awareness: It encourages a deeper understanding of your eating habits, allowing you to make conscious choices aligned with your health goals.

Understanding Intuitive Eating:

Intuitive eating is a philosophy developed by Evelyn Tribole and Elyse Resch in the 1990s. It promotes a compassionate and non-diet approach to eating, centering on the belief that individuals are born with an innate ability to regulate their eating patterns based on their body's cues.

Principles of Intuitive Eating:

1. Reject the Diet Mentality: Intuitive eating begins by letting go of the diet mentality and the pursuit of quick-fix weight loss solutions.

2. Honor Hunger: Intuitive eaters learn to respect their natural hunger signals, eating when they're hungry and stopping when they're full.

3. Make Peace with Food: All foods are allowed, and there are no "good" or "bad" foods. Intuitive eating encourages a balanced and non-restrictive approach to eating.

4. Challenge the Food Police: Intuitive eaters challenge the inner critic that enforces food rules and judgments about eating choices.

5. Respect Fullness: Tuning into the body's signals of fullness helps individuals avoid overeating and respect their body's limits.

6. Discover Satisfaction: Intuitive eating encourages finding pleasure and satisfaction in food, allowing the enjoyment of eating to be a central focus.

7. Cope with Emotions Without Using Food: This principle emphasizes finding

alternative ways to cope with emotions and stress instead of turning to food.

8. Respect Your Body: Intuitive eating promotes self-acceptance and body positivity, recognizing that bodies come in all shapes and sizes.

9. Exercise for Enjoyment: Instead of viewing exercise as a means to burn calories, intuitive eating encourages physical activity for the joy of movement.

Benefits of Intuitive Eating:

1. Improved Body Image: Intuitive eating fosters a positive relationship with one's body, promoting self-acceptance and body positivity.

2. Reduced Emotional Eating: By addressing emotional eating patterns, intuitive eating helps individuals develop healthier coping mechanisms.

3. Freedom from Dieting: Intuitive eating liberates individuals from the dieting cycle, allowing them to break free from restrictive eating patterns.

4. Sustainable Weight Management: Many intuitive eaters find that they naturally settle at a weight that is healthy for their body without restrictive dieting.

5. Enhanced Psychological Well-Being: Intuitive eating can reduce anxiety and guilt related to food, leading to improved emotional well-being.

Practical Tips for Mindful and Intuitive Eating:

1. Eat Without Distractions: Avoid eating in front of screens or while multitasking. Focus solely on your meal.

2. Chew Slowly: Take your time to chew each bite thoroughly, savoring the flavors.

3. Listen to Your Body: Pay attention to hunger and fullness cues. Eat when you're hungry and stop when you're satisfied.

4. Question Food Rules: Challenge any restrictive or rigid food rules you may have adopted over the years.

5. Embrace All Foods: Allow yourself to enjoy a wide variety of foods without judgment.

6. Practice Self-Compassion: Be kind to yourself, especially when facing challenges or setbacks in your eating journey.

Mindful eating and intuitive eating offer profound and sustainable approaches to nourishing both the body and soul. They invite individuals to embrace a non-diet mentality, cultivate self-compassion, and develop a more positive relationship with food. By fostering mindfulness, respecting body cues, and embracing all foods without judgment, these practices empower individuals to reclaim their innate wisdom and find balance, satisfaction, and joy in their eating experiences. Whether you're seeking a healthier relationship with food, improved well-being, or a more positive body image, mindful eating and intuitive eating provide a transformative path towards a more fulfilling and nourished life.

7.2 Emotional Eating and Coping Strategies

Emotions and eating are deeply intertwined. For many individuals, food serves not only as nourishment for the body but also as a source of comfort, celebration, and solace for the soul.

However, when emotional eating becomes a predominant coping mechanism, it can lead to weight gain and hinder weight loss efforts. In this comprehensive guide, we will explore the complex phenomenon of emotional eating, delve into its causes and consequences, and provide a multitude of effective coping strategies to help individuals regain control over their eating habits and ultimately support their weight loss goals.

Understanding Emotional Eating:

Emotional eating, often referred to as stress eating or comfort eating, involves using food as a means to manage and soothe emotional distress or discomfort. It is not necessarily driven by physical hunger but rather by emotional triggers such as stress, sadness, boredom, loneliness, or even happiness.

Common Triggers for Emotional Eating:

1. Stress: High-stress levels can lead to cravings for comfort foods like sweets, salty snacks, or high-calorie treats.

2. Sadness or Depression: Emotional distress may prompt individuals to seek solace in food to temporarily lift their mood.

3. Boredom: Feelings of monotony or lack of stimulation can lead to mindless snacking or overeating out of sheer boredom.

4. Loneliness: Loneliness or feelings of isolation may drive individuals to turn to food for companionship or distraction.

5. Celebration: Even positive emotions like happiness and celebration can trigger overindulgence in special occasions and gatherings.

The Consequences of Emotional Eating:

Both on one's physical and emotional wellbeing, emotional eating can have serious repercussions:

1. Weight Gain: Relying on food to deal with emotions on a regular basis might result in calorie overconsumption and weight gain.

2. Guilt and Shame: Following emotional eating episodes, people may feel guilty or ashamed, which exacerbates their emotional suffering.

3. Emotional eating does not deal with the underlying reasons of emotional pain, leaving unresolved difficulties.

4. Cycle of Emotional Eating: Emotional eating has the potential to spiral out of

control, increasing both one's emotional pain and dependence on food.

Effective Coping Strategies for Emotional Eating:

1. Mindfulness Meditation: Practicing mindfulness techniques can help individuals become more aware of their emotions and reduce impulsive eating behaviors.

2. Emotion Journaling: Keeping an emotion journal to track emotional triggers for eating can provide valuable insights and help identify patterns.

3. Healthy Stress Management: Using practices like deep breathing, exercise, and relaxation to control your stress might help you feel less the urge to eat emotionally.

4. Create a Support Network: Sharing emotions and seeking support from friends, family, or a therapist can

provide healthier outlets for emotional expression.

5. Intuitive Eating: Learning to listen to one's body and eat in response to physical hunger rather than emotions can be a powerful strategy.

6. Distract and Delay: When the urge to emotionally eat strikes, distract yourself with a non-food activity, and delay eating for a set period. Often, the urge will pass.

7. Plan Meals and Snacks: Having structured meals and snacks throughout the day can help prevent mindless or emotional eating.

8. Healthy Food Swaps: Replace high-calorie comfort foods with healthier alternatives that still provide comfort without excess calories.

9. Seek Professional Assistance: Consulting with a therapist or counselor might be helpful if emotional eating develops into a recurring problem that interferes with weight loss efforts or has an impact on mental health.

The Role of Emotional Intelligence:

Emotional intelligence, the ability to recognize and manage one's own emotions, is a valuable asset in addressing emotional eating. Individuals with higher emotional intelligence can better identify emotional triggers for overeating and develop healthier coping mechanisms.

The Importance of Self-Compassion:

It's essential to approach the journey of overcoming emotional eating with self-compassion. Self-criticism and harsh judgment can perpetuate emotional eating patterns. Instead, practice self-kindness and acknowledge that setbacks are a natural part of change.

Emotional eating is a complex and common challenge on the path to weight loss and improved well-being. It is essential to recognize that emotions and food are intricately connected and that addressing emotional eating requires a multifaceted approach. By cultivating emotional awareness, developing healthy coping strategies, seeking support when needed, and practicing self-compassion, individuals can regain control over their eating habits and move toward a healthier, more balanced relationship with food. In the end, overcoming emotional eating involves more than just weight loss; it also entails establishing higher emotional and psychological well-being, enabling people to lead lives that are more meaningful and empowered.

7.3 Visualization and Affirmations

Weight loss is not just a physical journey; it's a mental and emotional one as well. While diet and exercise play pivotal roles in shedding pounds, the power of the mind should not be underestimated. Visualization and affirmations are two potent tools that can help individuals overcome mental barriers, stay motivated, and achieve their weight loss goals. In this comprehensive guide, we will delve deep into the world of visualization and affirmations, exploring their principles, techniques, benefits, and how they can be harnessed to reshape your mindset and, ultimately, your body.

Understanding the Power of Visualization:

Visualization, also known as mental imagery, is a practice that involves creating detailed mental images of desired outcomes. It's a process of mentally rehearsing a scenario in vivid detail before it happens. In the context of weight loss, visualization can be a powerful tool for shaping a positive self-image, reinforcing motivation, and overcoming obstacles.

Principles of Effective Visualization:

1. Clarity: The more detailed and clear your mental images are, the more effective they become. Imagine yourself in your desired body with as much specificity as possible.

2. Emotion: Engage your emotions while visualizing. Feel the excitement, happiness, and pride associated with achieving your weight loss goals.

3. Consistency: Regular practice is essential. Incorporate visualization into your daily routine to reinforce your commitment.

4. Belief: Visualize with unwavering belief in your ability to achieve your goals. Self-doubt can undermine the effectiveness of visualization.

Visualization Techniques for Weight Loss:

1. Positive Body Image: Close your eyes and visualize your body as you want it to be. Picture yourself feeling confident and happy in your own skin.

2. Healthy Habits: Visualize yourself engaging in healthy habits like mindful eating and regular exercise. See yourself making nutritious choices effortlessly.

3. Overcoming Challenges: When faced with obstacles or cravings, mentally

rehearse how you will overcome them with determination and willpower.

4. Goal Achievement: Imagine the moment of reaching your weight loss goal. Feel the sense of accomplishment and celebrate your success.

The Power of Affirmations:

Affirmations are positive statements that reflect your desired goals and beliefs. When used consistently, affirmations can reprogram your subconscious mind, replacing self-limiting beliefs with empowering ones. In the context of weight loss, affirmations can boost self-esteem, motivation, and confidence.

Principles of Effective Affirmations:

Positive and Present Tense: Phrase your affirmations in the present tense, as if you've already achieved your goal. Keep them positive and avoid negative language.

1. Repetition: Consistently repeat your affirmations daily, multiple times if possible. Repetition helps embed them in your subconscious mind.

2. Belief: Believe in the truth of your affirmations. Doubt can undermine their effectiveness.

3. Emotion: Say your affirmations with genuine emotion. Feel the positivity and empowerment behind each statement.

Affirmations for Weight Loss:

"I'm on a path to a happier, healthier version of myself."

"My body is getting healthier and stronger every day."
"I make healthy food choices that fuel both my body and mind."
"I make thoughtful decisions and am in control of my eating habits."
"I effortlessly and gracefully release excess weight."
"I accept and love myself at every stage of my journey."
"I am deserving of a healthy, vibrant body."
"I am dedicated to my physical and mental well-being."
"I have the capability to overcome any obstacle in my path."
"I am appreciative of the advancement I am making."

Combining Visualization and Affirmations to supercharge your weight loss efforts, combine visualization and affirmations. Here's how:

1. Create a Visualization Script: Develop a detailed script that incorporates your affirmations. Imagine yourself actively living out your affirmations in your mental imagery.

2. Practice Mindfulness: Before engaging in visualization, take a few moments to clear your mind and center yourself. Deep breathing can help you enter a state of relaxation.

3. Visualization Sessions: Set aside dedicated time for visualization sessions. Find a quiet, comfortable space where you won't be interrupted.

4. Engage Your Senses: In your visualization, engage all your senses. Feel the emotions, hear the sounds, and see the vivid details of your desired outcomes.

5. Repeat Affirmations: As you visualize, repeat your chosen affirmations to

reinforce the positive beliefs associated with your goals.

Benefits of Visualization and Affirmations for Weight Loss:

1. Increased Motivation: Visualization and affirmations keep your goals at the forefront of your mind, motivating you to stay on track.

2. Enhanced Self-Confidence: These practices boost self-esteem and confidence, helping you believe in your ability to succeed.

3. Stress Reduction: Regular visualization can reduce stress and anxiety, which can often lead to emotional eating.

4. Positive Mindset: Over time, visualization and affirmations can help you cultivate a more positive and optimistic mindset.

5. Behavior Modification: These techniques can facilitate healthier behaviors and choices aligned with your weight loss goals.

Visualization and affirmations are powerful tools that can transform your mindset and support your weight loss journey. By consistently practicing these techniques, you can reprogram your subconscious mind, boost self-belief, and stay motivated on the path to achieving your weight loss goals. Remember that while visualization and affirmations are valuable, they are most effective when complemented by healthy eating habits and regular physical activity. When used in harmony with a holistic approach, these mental tools can help you harness the power of your mind to transform your body and lead you toward a healthier, happier you.

7.4 Meditation and stress reduction

In the quest for weight loss, the focus often falls squarely on diet and exercise. While these are undeniably crucial components, another, often underestimated factor plays an equally significant role: stress. Stress, both chronic and acute, can sabotage even the most well-structured weight loss plans. This comprehensive guide explores the intricate connection between meditation, stress reduction, and weight loss. By understanding the profound influence of stress on our bodies and the transformative power of meditation, you can unlock the hidden potential for lasting, successful weight management.

The Stress-Weight Connection:

To appreciate the impact of stress on weight, it's essential to grasp how our bodies respond to stressors. When we encounter stress, our bodies release hormones, including cortisol, often referred to as the "stress hormone." While cortisol is essential for survival, chronic stress can lead to persistently elevated levels, which can wreak havoc on our health and weight in several ways:

1. Cravings for High-Calorie Foods: Chronic stress can trigger cravings for comfort foods, often high in sugar and unhealthy fats, leading to overeating and weight gain.

2. Abdominal Fat Accumulation: Elevated cortisol levels are associated with fat storage, particularly around the abdominal area, which is linked to various health risks.

3. Emotional Eating: Stress often leads to emotional eating, where individuals depend on food as a coping mechanism,

leading to higher calorie level and increased weight.

4. Disrupted Sleep: Stress can disrupt sleep patterns, affecting the quality and duration of rest, which is essential for weight management.

5. Metabolic Changes: Chronic stress can lead to metabolic changes that make it harder to lose weight.

The Role of Meditation in Stress Reduction:

Meditation is a centuries-old practice that has gained recognition in recent years for its remarkable ability to reduce stress and promote overall well-being. At its core, meditation involves focused attention, mindfulness, and deep relaxation. When practiced regularly, meditation can mitigate the adverse effects of stress on the body and mind.

Benefits of Meditation for Stress Reduction:

1. Cortisol Reduction: Meditation has been shown to lower cortisol levels, reducing the physiological impact of stress.

2. Enhanced Emotional Regulation: Meditation improves emotional resilience and the ability to manage stress-inducing emotions without turning to food.

3. Improved Sleep: Regular meditation can lead to more restful and restorative sleep, which is crucial for weight loss and overall health.

4. Mindful Eating: Meditation fosters mindful eating, helping individuals become more attuned to hunger and fullness cues, making it easier to control portion sizes.

5. Stress Resilience: Meditation brings about stress resilience, helping individuals to cope better with life's challenges without turning to emotional eating.

Types of Meditation for Stress Reduction:

1. Mindfulness Meditation: This practice involves non-judgmental awareness of the present moment, which can help reduce stress and emotional eating.

2. Transcendental Meditation: Transcendental meditation employs the repetition of a mantra to induce a deep state of relaxation and reduce stress.

3. Yoga Nidra: A form of guided meditation, Yoga Nidra promotes deep relaxation and can be especially helpful for improving sleep.

4. Focused Attention Meditation: In this practice, individuals concentrate their attention on a specific object or thought, helping redirect the mind from stressors.

5. Loving-Kindness Meditation: This meditation focuses on cultivating feelings of compassion and love, which can counteract stress and promote emotional well-being.

Incorporating Meditation into Your Weight Loss Journey:

1. Set Realistic Goals: Begin with a manageable meditation routine that aligns with your lifestyle. As little as 10-15 minutes a day can yield benefits.

2. Create a Sacred Space: Designate a quiet, comfortable space for meditation, free from distractions.

3. Consistency is Key: Establish a regular meditation practice. Consistency amplifies the benefits over time.

4. Mindful Eating: Incorporate mindfulness into your meals. Pay attention to each bite, savoring the flavors and textures.

5. Combine with Physical Activity: Pair meditation with physical activity, such as yoga or mindful walking, for holistic stress management.

Real-Life Success Stories:

Numerous individuals have experienced transformative weight loss and overall well-being through the integration of meditation and stress reduction techniques into their lives. These success stories highlight the profound impact of managing stress on weight management:

Sarah, 35: Sarah battled emotional eating for years. Through mindfulness meditation, she learned to identify her emotional triggers and developed healthier coping mechanisms. As a result, she lost 30 pounds and felt more in control of her eating habits.

Michael, 42: Michael's demanding job led to chronic stress and weight gain. He incorporated transcendental meditation into his daily routine, which reduced his stress levels and improved his sleep. Over the course of a year, he lost 50 pounds.

In the journey toward successful weight loss, stress reduction through meditation is a game-changer. By addressing the physiological and psychological impacts of stress, meditation empowers individuals to regain control over their eating habits, reduce emotional eating, and achieve sustainable weight management.

Remember that meditation is not a quick fix but a valuable tool for long-term well-being. When paired with a balanced diet and regular physical activity, meditation can unlock the hidden potential within you, helping you achieve your weight loss goals while fostering a deeper sense of inner peace and vitality.

Chapter 8: Combining Strategies for Success

8.1 Creating a Personalized Weight Loss Plan

Embarking on a weight loss journey can be both exciting and daunting. While there's an abundance of advice and diets available, finding a personalized approach that suits your unique needs, preferences, and lifestyle is key to achieving sustainable results. In this comprehensive discussion, we will explore the steps to create a personalized weight loss plan that empowers you to reach your goals and maintain a healthier lifestyle.

Step 1: Define Your Goals and Motivation

Before diving into any weight loss plan, it's essential to define your goals and motivation. Ask yourself:

- What are your specific weight loss goals?

- Why do you want to lose weight?

- What motivates you to make a change?

Understanding your goals and motivations will provide you with a clear direction and help you stay committed throughout your journey.

Step 2: Assess Your Current Lifestyle

Take an honest look at your current lifestyle, including your eating habits, physical activity level, sleep patterns, and stress management. Reflect on:

- Your typical daily diet.

- How often you engage in physical activity.

- Your sleep duration and quality.

- How you manage stress.

Identifying areas where you can make improvements will guide your personalized plan.

Step 3: Consult a Healthcare Professional

Before making significant dietary or exercise changes, consult with a healthcare professional, such as a doctor or registered dietitian. They can assess your overall health, any underlying medical conditions, and provide guidance tailored to your needs and safety.

Step 4: Set Realistic and Sustainable Goals

Ensure your weight loss goals are realistic and sustainable. Rapid or extreme weight loss approaches may not lead to long-term success and can be detrimental to your health. Aim for gradual, steady progress.

Step 5: Create a Balanced Diet Plan

Design a balanced diet plan that aligns with your preferences and dietary requirements. Focus on the following principles:

- Portion Control: To properly limit calorie consumption, pay attention to portion sizes.

- To ensure a wide range of nutrients, include a variety of foods in your diet.

295

- Give whole, unprocessed foods like fruits, vegetables, lean meats, whole grains, and healthy fats top priority.

- Hydration: To boost your metabolism and general health, drink enough water throughout the day.

Customize your meal plan in Step 6

Make your meal plan specifically for your requirements and preferences. Consider elements like:

- Food allergies or intolerances.

- Cultural or dietary restrictions.

- Meal timing and frequency.

- Personalizing your meal plan will make it more sustainable and enjoyable.

Step 7: Implement Mindful Eating

To have a healthier relationship with food, practice mindful eating. Be mindful of your hunger and fullness cues, enjoy every bite, and keep distractions to a minimum while eating. By using this strategy, overeating and emotional eating can be avoided.

Step 8: Establish an Exercise Program

Make regular exercise a part of your regimen. Whether you prefer cycling, swimming, dancing, or strolling, pick an activity you enjoy. Aim for a balance of flexibility, strength training, and cardiovascular activity.

Step 9: Set Up a Support System

Share your weight loss goals with friends or family members who can provide support and encouragement. You might also consider joining a support group or working with a personal trainer or nutritionist for added guidance and accountability.

Step 10: Monitor Your Progress

Keep track of your progress using various methods, such as:

- Regular weigh-ins.

- Body measurements (waist, hips, etc.).

- Food journals to record your meals and snacks.

- Exercise logs to track your workouts.

Monitoring your progress allows you to make adjustments as needed and celebrate your successes.

Step 11: Be Patient and Persistent

Weight loss is not always linear, and you may encounter plateaus or setbacks along the way. Be patient with yourself and stay persistent, focusing on the long-term health benefits of your journey.

Step 12: Seek Professional Guidance as Needed

If you encounter challenges or if your weight loss stalls, don't hesitate to seek professional guidance. A registered dietitian or personal trainer can provide tailored advice and help you navigate obstacles.

Step 13: Embrace Lifestyle Changes

Ultimately, successful weight loss is about making sustainable lifestyle changes. Rather than viewing your plan as a temporary diet, think of it as a long-term commitment to your health and well-being.

Creating a personalized weight loss plan is a crucial step toward achieving your goals and improving your overall health. By defining your objectives, assessing your current lifestyle, seeking professional guidance, and implementing sustainable changes, you can develop a plan that aligns with your unique needs and preferences. Remember that weight loss is a journey, and the key to success lies in patience, persistence, and a commitment to long-term lifestyle changes.

8.2 Tracking Progress and Adjusting Strategies

Embarking on a weight loss journey is an endeavor filled with determination and commitment. To achieve your goals successfully and maintain a healthier lifestyle, it's essential to not only start but also continue tracking your progress and making adjustments as needed. In this comprehensive discussion, we will explore the significance of tracking weight loss progress and how to adapt your strategies for long-term success.

The Importance of Tracking Progress

Effective weight loss isn't just about shedding pounds; it's also about improving overall health and well-being. Tracking your progress provides several benefits:

1. Accountability: Regularly monitoring your weight, measurements, and habits keeps you accountable to your goals.

2. Motivation: Seeing positive changes over time can boost your motivation and reinforce your commitment to the journey.

3. Identifying Trends: Tracking allows you to identify trends in your progress, helping you understand what works and what doesn't.

4. Early Intervention: Recognizing plateaus or setbacks early enables you to take action to overcome them.

5. Celebrating Achievements: Acknowledging and celebrating your achievements, even small ones, can provide a sense of accomplishment and encouragement.

Methods of Tracking Progress

There are several effective methods for tracking weight loss progress:

1. Weighing Scale: Regular weigh-ins (e.g., once a week) provide a quantitative measure of your progress. Keep in mind that weight can fluctuate daily due to factors like hydration and digestion, so focus on trends over time.

2. Body Measurements: Taking measurements of key areas like your waist, hips, chest, and thighs can reveal changes in body composition, even if the scale doesn't budge.

3. Progress Photos: Comparing before-and-after photos can provide visual evidence of your transformation.

4. Food Diary: Keeping a food diary helps you monitor your eating habits, identify potential trouble spots, and make necessary adjustments.

5. Exercise Logs: Recording your physical activity helps you ensure you're meeting your fitness goals and staying consistent with your workouts.

6. Health Markers: Consider tracking other health markers such as blood pressure, cholesterol levels, and blood sugar, as these can provide a more comprehensive picture of your health.

7. Daily Routine: You can also track daily habits like sleep duration and stress management, as these factors can impact weight loss progress.

How to Adjust Your Strategies

Adaptability is a crucial aspect of successful weight loss. If you encounter challenges or stagnation in your progress, it's time to consider making adjustments:

1. Review Your Diet:

- Calorie Intake: Are you consuming the right number of calories for your goals? Adjust as needed to create a calorie deficit.

- Macronutrient Balance: Ensure you have a balanced intake of carbohydrates, proteins, and fats.
- Nutrient Density: Focus on nutrient-dense foods to meet your nutritional needs.

- Meal Timing: Experiment with meal timing and frequency to see if it impacts your appetite and energy levels.

2. Reevaluate Exercise Routine:

- Intensity: Adjust the intensity of your workouts to challenge your body and prevent adaptation.

- Variety: Incorporate different exercises and activities to keep things interesting and target various muscle groups.

- Frequency: Assess whether you need to increase or decrease the frequency of your workouts.

3. Monitor Habits:

- Sleep: Ensure you're getting adequate rest, as sleep plays a crucial role in weight management.

- Stress Management: Implement stress-reduction techniques, such as mindfulness or meditation, if stress is affecting your progress.

- Hydration: Stay properly hydrated, as thirst can sometimes be mistaken for hunger.

4. Seek Professional Guidance:

- Registered Dietitian: Consult with a registered dietitian to assess your dietary habits and receive personalized recommendations.

- Personal Trainer: A personal trainer can help you design an effective exercise plan and ensure you're using proper form.

- Medical Professional: If you encounter significant challenges or health concerns, seek guidance from a medical professional.

5. Be Patient and Realistic:

Weight loss doesn't always occur at a consistent rate. Plateaus are common, but they can be overcome with persistence and adaptation.
Set realistic expectations and focus on long-term health rather than quick fixes.

6. Stay Consistent:

Consistency is key to long-term success. Even if progress is slow, maintaining healthy habits is essential.

7. Celebrate Achievements:

Acknowledge and celebrate your achievements along the way, whether it's reaching a specific weight, achieving a fitness milestone, or maintaining a healthier lifestyle.

Tracking weight loss progress and adjusting your strategies as needed are integral parts of a successful and sustainable weight loss journey. Regular monitoring provides accountability, motivation, and valuable insights into your progress. When faced with challenges or stagnation, don't get discouraged; instead, use these moments as opportunities to fine-tune your approach and make positive changes. Remember that weight loss is a journey, and the path to success is characterized by adaptability, patience, and a commitment to long-term health and well-being.

8.3 Breaking Through Plateaus

Embarking on a weight loss journey can be an exhilarating experience filled with initial progress and newfound motivation. However, it's not uncommon to encounter plateaus along the way—those frustrating periods where your weight seems to have hit a roadblock, refusing to budge despite your continued efforts. These plateaus can be disheartening and test your resolve, but they are also crucial moments for growth and learning. In this comprehensive discussion, we will explore the reasons behind weight loss plateaus and provide you with a toolbox of effective strategies to break through them and continue your journey toward your weight loss goals.

Understanding Weight Loss Plateaus

Before diving into strategies to overcome plateaus, it's essential to understand what they are and why they occur. A weight loss plateau refers to a phase during your weight loss journey when your progress comes to a seemingly grinding halt. You might notice that the numbers on the scale haven't budged, or your body measurements have remained stagnant for several weeks. Plateaus are a natural part of the weight loss process, and they happen for various reasons:

1. Metabolic Adaptation: As you lose weight, your body's metabolic rate can decrease, meaning it burns fewer calories at rest than when you started your journey. This can reduce the calorie

deficit that was once driving your weight loss.

2. Reduced Calorie Deficit: As your body weight decreases, the same caloric deficit that led to initial weight loss may no longer be sufficient to promote further weight loss. Your body may have adapted to this new calorie intake.

3. Exercise Adaptation: Your body can become more efficient at performing the exercises you regularly engage in, which can reduce the number of calories burned during workouts.

4. Water Retention: Temporary water weight gain can obscure your true fat loss progress on the scale, especially if your body is retaining water due to factors like increased sodium intake or inflammation.

5. Psychological Factors: Plateaus can also be influenced by psychological

factors such as stress, lack of motivation, or inconsistent adherence to your plan. Emotional eating or mindless snacking can sometimes creep in during these periods.

Effective Strategies for Breaking Through Plateaus

Breaking through a weight loss plateau requires a multifaceted approach that addresses both dietary and lifestyle factors. Here are several strategies to consider:

Reassess Your Caloric Intake:

1. Recalculate Maintenance Calories: Over time, your maintenance calorie level may have changed due to weight loss. Recalculate your maintenance calories and adjust your daily intake accordingly.

2. Reduce Caloric Intake: Slightly reduce your daily calorie intake to create a new, sustainable calorie deficit. Avoid drastic reductions, as they can be counterproductive and unsustainable.

Increase Physical Activity:

1. Change Your Routine: Modify your exercise routine by incorporating new activities or intensifying your workouts to challenge your body.

2. Strength Training: Include strength training exercises to build lean muscle mass, which can boost your metabolism and help you break through plateaus.

3. HIIT Workouts: High-Intensity Interval Training (HIIT) can be an effective way to increase calorie burn and overcome plateaus by introducing variety and intensity into your workouts.

Practice Mindful Eating:

1.   Food   Quality: Emphasize nutrient-dense foods such as fruits, vegetables, lean proteins, and whole grains to support your overall health and weight loss.

2. Portion Control: Be mindful of portion sizes to avoid overeating, especially during meals. Smaller, balanced portions can help regulate calorie intake.

3. Avoid Mindless Snacking: Limit or eliminate mindless snacking and emotional eating by identifying triggers and finding alternative coping strategies, such as engaging in a hobby or going for a walk when cravings strike.

Stay Hydrated:

1. Water Intake: Ensure you are drinking an   adequate   amount   of   water

throughout the day. Proper hydration can help with satiety and reduce water retention, potentially revealing your true weight loss progress.
Monitor Your Progress:

2. Body Measurements: In addition to tracking your weight on the scale, measure key areas of your body like your waist, hips, and chest. Sometimes, even when the scale doesn't move, you're still making positive changes in body composition.

3. Progress Photos: Take regular progress photos to visually assess your transformation. Visual evidence can be motivating and show changes that might not be reflected on the scale.

Prioritize Sleep and Stress Management:

1. Sleep Quality: Aim for 7-9 hours of quality sleep per night to support overall

health and metabolic function. A well-rested body is better equipped to manage weight.

2. Stress Reduction: Implement stress-reduction techniques such as meditation, yoga, or deep breathing exercises to manage stress levels. High stress can lead to hormonal changes that can hinder weight loss.

Be Patient and Persistent:

1. Set Realistic Expectations: Understand that plateaus are a normal part of the weight loss process, and weight loss may not always be linear. Set realistic expectations and focus on long-term progress rather than quick fixes.

2. Stay Consistent: Consistency in your dietary and exercise habits is crucial to overcoming plateaus. Even when

progress seems slow, maintaining healthy habits is essential.

Seek Professional Guidance:

1. Registered Dietitian: Consult with a registered dietitian for personalized advice and dietary adjustments based on your specific circumstances and goals.

2. Fitness Trainer: A fitness trainer can help you modify your workout routine for better results and ensure you're using proper form to avoid injuries.

3. Medical Professional: If you experience prolonged plateaus or have health concerns, consult a medical professional for a thorough evaluation and guidance.

Consider a Diet Break:

1. Intermittent Dieting: Incorporate intermittent dieting phases where you

briefly increase calorie intake to maintenance levels. This can help mitigate metabolic adaptation and break through plateaus.
Review and Adjust Goals:

2. Reevaluate Goals: Periodically review your weight loss goals and adjust them if necessary. Consider focusing on non-scale victories, such as improved energy levels, better sleep, or increased fitness capabilities, to maintain motivation.

Weight loss plateaus are a common and expected part of the weight loss journey. While they can be disheartening, they are also opportunities for personal growth and learning. By understanding the factors that contribute to plateaus and implementing a combination of dietary and lifestyle strategies, you can effectively break through these obstacles and continue progressing toward your weight loss goals. It's important to remember that weight loss is a marathon, not a sprint, and patience, adaptability, and consistency are key to achieving and maintaining a healthier you. Embrace plateaus as opportunities for growth, stay committed to your journey, and celebrate each milestone along the way.

8.4 Setting Realistic Goals

Embarking on a weight loss journey can be an exhilarating experience filled with initial progress and newfound motivation. However, it's not uncommon to encounter plateaus along the way—those frustrating periods where your weight seems to have hit a roadblock, refusing to budge despite your continued efforts. These plateaus can be disheartening and test your resolve, but they are also crucial moments for growth and learning. In this discussion, we will explore the reasons behind weight loss plateaus and provide you with effective strategies to break through them and continue your journey toward your weight loss goals.

Understanding Weight Loss Plateaus

Before diving into strategies to overcome plateaus, it's essential to understand what they are and why they occur. A weight loss plateau refers to a phase during your weight loss journey when your progress comes to a seemingly grinding halt. You might notice that the numbers on the scale haven't budged, or your body measurements have remained stagnant for several weeks. Plateaus are a natural part of the weight loss process, and they happen for various reasons:

1. Metabolic Adaptation: As you lose weight, your body's metabolic rate can decrease, meaning it burns fewer calories at rest than when you started

your journey. This can reduce the calorie deficit that was once driving your weight loss.

2. Reduced Calorie Deficit: As your body weight decreases, the same caloric deficit that led to initial weight loss may no longer be sufficient to promote further weight loss. Your body may have adapted to this new calorie intake.

3. Exercise Adaptation: Your body can become more efficient at performing the exercises you regularly engage in, which can reduce the number of calories burned during workouts.

4. Water Retention: Temporary water weight gain can obscure your true fat loss progress on the scale, especially if your body is retaining water due to factors like increased sodium intake or inflammation.

5. Psychological Factors: Plateaus can also be influenced by psychological factors such as stress, lack of motivation, or inconsistent adherence to your plan. Emotional eating or mindless snacking can sometimes creep in during these periods.

Effective Strategies for Breaking Through Plateaus

Breaking through a weight loss plateau requires a multifaceted approach that addresses both dietary and lifestyle factors. Here are several strategies to consider:

1. Reassess Your Caloric Intake:

Recalculate Maintenance Calories: Over time, your maintenance calorie level may have changed due to weight loss. Recalculate your maintenance calories and adjust your daily intake accordingly.

Reduce Caloric Intake: Slightly reduce your daily calorie intake to create a new, sustainable calorie deficit. Avoid drastic reductions, as they can be counterproductive and unsustainable.

2. Increase Physical Activity:

Change Your Routine: Modify your exercise routine by incorporating new activities or intensifying your workouts to challenge your body.

Strength Training: Include strength training exercises to build lean muscle mass, which can boost your metabolism and help you break through plateaus.

HIIT Workouts: High-Intensity Interval Training (HIIT) can be an effective way to increase calorie burn and overcome plateaus by introducing variety and intensity into your workouts.

3. Practice Mindful Eating:

Food Quality: Emphasize nutrient-dense foods such as fruits, vegetables, lean proteins, and whole grains to support your overall health and weight loss.

Portion Control: Be mindful of portion sizes to avoid overeating, especially during meals. Smaller, balanced portions can help regulate calorie intake.

Avoid Mindless Snacking: Limit or eliminate mindless snacking and emotional eating by identifying triggers and finding alternative coping strategies, such as engaging in a hobby or going for a walk when cravings strike.

4. Stay Hydrated:

Water Intake: Ensure you are drinking an adequate amount of water throughout the day. Proper hydration can help with satiety and reduce water retention, potentially revealing your true weight loss progress.

5. Monitor Your Progress:

Body Measurements: In addition to tracking your weight on the scale, measure key areas of your body like your waist, hips, and chest. Sometimes, even when the scale doesn't move, you're still making positive changes in body composition.

Progress Photos: Take regular progress photos to visually assess your transformation. Visual evidence can be motivating and show changes that might not be reflected on the scale.

6. Prioritize Sleep and Stress Management:

Sleep Quality: Aim for 7-9 hours of quality sleep per night to support overall health and metabolic function. A well-rested body is better equipped to manage weight.

Stress Reduction: Implement stress-reduction techniques such as meditation, yoga, or deep breathing exercises to manage stress levels. High stress can lead to hormonal changes that can hinder weight loss.

7. Be Patient and Persistent:

Set Realistic Expectations: Understand that plateaus are a normal part of the weight loss process, and weight loss may not always be linear. Set realistic expectations and focus on long-term progress rather than quick fixes.

Stay Consistent: Consistency in your dietary and exercise habits is crucial to overcoming plateaus. Even when progress seems slow, maintaining healthy habits is essential.

8. Seek Professional Guidance:

Registered Dietitian: Consult with a registered dietitian for personalized advice and dietary adjustments based on your specific circumstances and goals.

Fitness Trainer: A fitness trainer can help you modify your workout routine for better results and ensure you're using proper form to avoid injuries.

Medical Professional: If you experience prolonged plateaus or have health concerns, consult a medical professional for a thorough evaluation and guidance.

9. Consider a Diet Break:

Intermittent Dieting: Incorporate intermittent dieting phases where you briefly increase calorie intake to maintenance levels. This can help mitigate metabolic adaptation and break through plateaus.

Weight loss plateaus are a common and expected part of the weight loss journey. While they can be disheartening, they are also opportunities for personal growth and learning. By understanding the factors that contribute to plateaus and implementing a combination of dietary and lifestyle strategies, you can effectively break through these obstacles and continue progressing toward your weight loss goals. It's important to remember that weight loss is a marathon, not a sprint, and patience, adaptability, and consistency are key to achieving and maintaining a healthier you. Embrace plateaus as opportunities for growth, stay committed to your journey, and celebrate each milestone along the way.

Chapter 9: Maintaining Your Weight Loss

9.1 Transitioning to Maintenance Mode

Congratulations! You've made significant progress in your weight loss journey and achieved your desired weight loss goals. Now, you're at a pivotal point in your wellness journey: the transition to maintenance mode. This phase is just as crucial as the weight loss phase, as it involves maintaining your achievements and establishing sustainable habits that will keep you healthy and balanced in the long term. In this comprehensive discussion, we will explore the importance of transitioning to maintenance mode, the strategies to make this transition successful, and how to ensure that you continue enjoying a healthy and fulfilling life while keeping those extra pounds off.

Why Transition to Maintenance Mode?

Transitioning to maintenance mode signifies a shift from the active weight loss phase to maintaining your new healthy weight. It is a critical step for several reasons:

1. Sustainability: Prolonged periods of calorie restriction and intense exercise may not be sustainable in the long run. Transitioning to maintenance mode allows you to establish a balanced and sustainable lifestyle.

2. Metabolic Health: Rapid weight loss can sometimes lead to metabolic changes. By transitioning to maintenance mode, you give your body time to adapt to your new weight and maintain a healthy metabolism.

3. Psychological Well-being: Constantly aiming for weight loss can be mentally exhausting. Transitioning to maintenance mode provides a mental break and shifts your focus toward maintaining your progress.

4. Long-Term Success: Maintaining weight loss is often more challenging than losing weight. Transitioning to maintenance mode helps you develop the skills and habits needed for long-term success.

Strategies for a Successful Transition

Transitioning to maintenance mode requires a thoughtful approach and a commitment to maintaining your healthy lifestyle. Here are some key strategies to ensure a successful transition:

1. Gradual Caloric Adjustment: Slowly increase your calorie intake to your maintenance level. This prevents sudden weight gain and allows your body to adjust gradually.

2. Monitor Your Weight: Keep an eye on your weight during the transition phase. If you notice a significant increase, adjust your calorie intake or exercise routine accordingly.

3. Stay Active: Continue with regular physical activity, but you may adjust your exercise routine to focus on fitness and strength rather than weight loss.

4. Mindful Eating: Maintain the healthy eating habits you developed during your weight loss journey. Focus on nutrient-dense foods and portion control.

5. Celebrate Achievements: Acknowledge and celebrate your

achievements. Reward yourself with non-food treats for reaching milestones in your maintenance journey.

6. Stay Accountable: Consider joining a support group or working with a registered dietitian or personal trainer to stay accountable and receive guidance during this phase.

7. Prepare for Challenges: Be aware that challenges may arise during maintenance mode, such as stress or special occasions. Develop strategies to address these challenges without derailing your progress.

8. Regular Check-Ins: Periodically assess your progress and make necessary adjustments to your maintenance plan. This ensures that you stay on track and can make corrections if needed.

Enjoying a Healthy and Fulfilling Life in Maintenance Mode

Maintenance mode doesn't mean a life of deprivation or constant vigilance. It's an opportunity to enjoy the benefits of a healthier lifestyle while maintaining your weight. Here's how to make the most of this phase:

1. Explore New Activities: Use your newfound fitness to explore new physical activities and hobbies that you enjoy. Whether it's hiking, dancing, or yoga, find activities that bring you joy.

2. Expand Your Culinary Horizons: Continue to experiment with healthy recipes and foods. Trying new cuisines and cooking techniques can make healthy eating exciting and enjoyable.

3. Set New Goals: Consider setting new fitness or wellness goals to keep yourself motivated. These goals could include

running a certain distance, mastering a new exercise, or even participating in a fitness event.

4. Mindful Living: Practice mindfulness in all aspects of life. Pay attention to your body's hunger and fullness cues, savor your meals, and be present in the moment.

5. Embrace Balance: Remember that occasional indulgences are part of a balanced life. Enjoy your favorite treats in moderation without guilt.

6. Support Network: Stay connected with friends and loved ones who support your healthy lifestyle. Share your successes and challenges with them.

Transitioning to maintenance mode is a significant achievement in your weight loss journey. It's a phase where you consolidate your hard-earned progress and focus on a sustainable, healthy lifestyle. By implementing the strategies outlined above and embracing a balanced, mindful approach to life, you can enjoy a fulfilling and healthy future while maintaining your weight loss success. Keep in mind that this journey is about more than just numbers on a scale—it's about your overall well-being and happiness.

9.2 Long-Term Healthy Habits

Achieving your weight loss goals is a remarkable accomplishment, but maintaining a healthy weight over the long term is equally important. It requires adopting sustainable habits that become an integral part of your lifestyle. In this comprehensive discussion, we will explore a range of long-term healthy weight loss habits that can help you not only shed excess pounds but also sustain your progress and enjoy a healthier, happier life.

Balanced Diet:

- Portion Control: Continue to monitor your portion sizes to prevent overeating. Use smaller plates and practice mindful eating.

- Nutrient-Dense Foods: Emphasize a diet rich in fruits, vegetables, lean proteins, whole grains, and healthy fats. These foods provide essential nutrients and support your overall health.

- Regular Meals: Establish a consistent meal schedule to regulate your metabolism and prevent excessive hunger, which can lead to unhealthy snacking.

Regular Physical Activity:

- Aerobic Exercise: Engage in regular aerobic activities like walking, jogging, swimming, or cycling. Aim for at least 150 minutes of moderate-intensity exercise per week.

- Strength Training: Include strength training exercises to build lean muscle mass, boost your metabolism, and improve overall fitness.
- Flexibility and Balance: Incorporate activities like yoga or Pilates to improve flexibility and balance, enhancing your overall physical well-being.

Hydration:

- Water Intake: Stay adequately hydrated by drinking plenty of water throughout the day. Proper hydration supports metabolism and overall health.

Mindful Eating:

- Listen to Your Body: Pay attention to hunger and fullness cues. Eat when you're hungry and stop when you're satisfied.

- Limit Distractions: Avoid eating in front of the TV or computer, which can lead to mindless overeating.

- Savor Your Food: Take time to enjoy your meals, savoring each bite. This can lead to greater satisfaction and reduced overconsumption.

Consistency and Routine:

- Consistent Schedule: Maintain a regular daily routine for meals, exercise, and sleep. Consistency can help regulate metabolism and reduce the risk of overeating.

Stress Management:

- Stress Reduction: Implement stress-reduction techniques such as meditation, deep breathing exercises, or mindfulness practices. High stress levels can lead to emotional eating and weight gain.

- Self-Care: Prioritize self-care activities that promote relaxation and well-being, such as taking baths, reading, or spending time in nature.

Quality Sleep:

- Sleep Hygiene: Ensure you get 7-9 hours of quality sleep per night. Poor sleep can disrupt hormones related to appetite and lead to weight gain.

Regular Health Check-Ups:

- Medical Evaluation: Schedule regular check-ups with your healthcare provider to monitor your overall health, including weight, blood pressure, and cholesterol levels.

- Consult a Dietitian: Consider consulting a registered dietitian for personalized dietary guidance and adjustments.

Positive Mindset:

- Self-Compassion: Be kind to yourself and practice self-compassion. Weight fluctuations are normal, and it's essential to maintain a positive relationship with your body.

- Set Realistic Goals: Set achievable and realistic goals that focus on overall well-being rather than just a number on the scale.

Support Network:

- Community: Stay connected with friends, family, or support groups who share your wellness goals. A supportive network can provide encouragement and accountability.

Plan Ahead:

- Meal Planning: Plan your meals and snacks in advance to make healthier choices readily available and reduce the temptation of less nutritious options.

- Fitness Schedule: Schedule your workouts and activities in advance to ensure they fit into your daily routine.

Celebrate Non-Scale Victories:

- Non-Scale Achievements: Celebrate accomplishments beyond the scale, such as improved energy levels, better sleep, increased fitness capabilities, or fitting into old clothes.

Flexibility and Moderation:

- Occasional Treats: Allow yourself occasional treats and indulgences. A flexible approach to your diet can help prevent feelings of deprivation.

Long-term healthy weight loss habits are the key to maintaining your progress and enjoying a balanced, fulfilling life. By adopting these habits and integrating them into your daily routine, you can continue to reap the benefits of your weight loss journey and ensure a happier, healthier future. Remember that sustainable weight management is about more than just a number on the scale—it's about nourishing your body, staying active, and nurturing your overall well-being.

9.3 Preventing Weight Regain

One of the most significant challenges in the weight loss journey is preventing weight regain after achieving your desired goals. Many people experience a relapse into old habits, resulting in the reacquisition of lost pounds. However, with the right strategies and a commitment to long-term success, you can maintain your hard-earned progress and avoid weight regain. In this comprehensive discussion, we will explore effective strategies to help you stay on track, overcome common obstacles, and enjoy a healthy, sustainable weight for life.

Maintain a Balanced Diet:

- Portion Control: Continue to practice portion control, using smaller plates and mindful eating techniques.

- Nutrient-Rich Foods: Prioritize whole, nutrient-dense foods that provide essential vitamins and minerals while promoting a sense of fullness.

Regular Physical Activity:

- Consistency: Stay consistent with your exercise routine, aiming for a mix of aerobic, strength training, and flexibility exercises.

- Set Goals: Set new fitness goals to keep your workouts interesting and challenging.

Mindful Eating:

- Listen to Your Body: Continue to pay attention to your body's hunger and fullness cues.

- Avoid Emotional Eating: Implement strategies to manage emotional eating, such as journaling or practicing stress-reduction techniques.

Stay Hydrated:

- Water Intake: Maintain proper hydration by drinking water throughout the day. Sometimes, thirst can be mistaken for hunger.

Regular Meal Schedule:

- Consistent Timing: Stick to a regular meal schedule to help regulate your metabolism and avoid skipped meals, which can lead to overeating later.

Manage Stress:

- Stress Reduction: Prioritize stress management techniques, such as meditation, yoga, or spending time in nature.

- Self-Care: Incorporate self-care activities that promote relaxation and well-being.

Quality Sleep:

- Sleep Hygiene: Continue to prioritize 7-9 hours of quality sleep per night, as inadequate sleep can disrupt hunger hormones.

Regular Health Check-Ups:

- Medical Evaluation: Schedule regular check-ups with your healthcare provider to monitor your overall health and address any emerging issues promptly.

Positive Mindset:

- Self-Compassion: Practice self-compassion and maintain a positive relationship with your body.

- Set Realistic Goals: Set achievable and realistic goals that focus on overall well-being.

Support Network:

- Stay Connected: Maintain your support network of friends, family, or support groups to provide encouragement and accountability.

Celebrate Non-Scale Victories:

- Non-Scale Achievements: Continue to celebrate accomplishments beyond the scale to reinforce your commitment to a healthy lifestyle.

Plan Ahead:

- Meal and Fitness Planning: Plan your meals and workouts in advance to ensure you make healthy choices and prioritize exercise.

Regular Self-Monitoring:

- Food Journal: Keep a food journal to track your eating habits and identify areas where improvement is needed.

- Regular Weigh-Ins: Periodically check your weight to catch any significant changes early.

Flexibility and Moderation:

- Occasional Treats: Allow yourself occasional treats and indulgences while maintaining overall moderation.

Seek Professional Support:

- Dietitian or Counselor: Consult with a registered dietitian or counselor if you find yourself struggling with old habits or emotional eating.

Preventing weight regain is an ongoing journey that requires dedication, mindfulness, and a commitment to long-term success. By incorporating these strategies into your daily life and embracing a holistic approach to your well-being, you can maintain your hard-earned progress, avoid relapse, and enjoy a healthy, sustainable weight for years to come. Remember that setbacks may occur, but with resilience and the right support system, you can overcome challenges and stay on the path to lifelong health and wellness.

Conclusion

In closing, your weight loss journey is a testament to your commitment to better health and well-being. It's not just about the numbers on the scale but about embracing a lifestyle that prioritizes your overall wellness. As you reflect on the knowledge and strategies you've acquired, remember that this journey is an ongoing commitment.

Take pride in your accomplishments, whether you've achieved your goals or are well on your way. Your efforts deserve recognition, and you should celebrate every milestone along the way.

Your journey is not finite; it's a continuous dedication to maintaining your progress and health. Sustainability and balance should be at the forefront of your choices.

Mindful eating, emotional well-being, regular physical activity, and a positive mindset are the cornerstones of your path forward. Practice self-compassion, stay connected with a supportive network, and appreciate the occasional indulgence in moderation.

Your health is an ongoing priority. Regular check-ups with healthcare professionals, dietitians, or counselors ensure that you continue on the right path.

Embrace personal growth and the positive changes you've experienced on your journey. Continue to set new goals and envision a future filled with health, happiness, and vitality.

Your journey is unique, and your potential is boundless. As you close this book, envision the vibrant and healthy life that awaits you. Your commitment to improving your life is inspiring, and I wish you lasting success, fulfillment, and well-being on your path to a healthier you.

Thank you for choosing this book as your companion on your weight loss journey.